PREIMPLANTATION DIAGNOSIS OF GENETIC DISEASES

A New Technique in Assisted Reproduction

PREIMPLANTATION DIAGNOSIS OF GENETIC DISEASES

A New Technique in Assisted Reproduction

EDITORS: YURY VERLINSKY
AND ANVER M. KULIEV
Reproductive Genetics Institute
Illinois Masonic Medical Center
Chicago, Illinois

WILEY-LISS
A JOHN WILEY & SONS, INC., PUBLICATION
New York • Chichester • Brisbane • Toronto • Singapore

Address All Inquiries to the Publisher
Wiley-Liss, Inc., 605 Third Avenue, New York, NY 10158-0012

Printed in the United States of America

While the authors, editors, and publisher believe that drug selection and dosage and the specifications and usage of equipment and devices, as set forth in this book, are in accord with current recommendations and practice at the time of publication, they accept no legal responsibility for any errors or omissions, and make no warranty, express or implied, with respect to material contained herein. In view of ongoing research, equipment modifications, changes in governmental regulations and the constant flow of information relating to drug therapy, drug reactions and the use of equipment and devices, the reader is urged to review and evaluate the information provided in the package insert or instructions or indications of dosage or usage and for added warnings and precautions.

For a description of the cover illustration please see page 59.

Library of Congress Cataloging-in-Publication Data

Preimplantation diagnosis of genetic diseases : a new technique in
assisted reproduction / edited by Yury Verlinsky, Anver M. Kuliev.
p. cm.
Includes bibliographical references and index.
ISBN 0-471-58824-5
1. Preimplantation genetic diagnosis. I. Verlinsky, Yury.
II. Kuliev, Anver M.
[DNLM: 1. Hereditary Diseases—diagnosis. 2. Preimplantation
Phase. 3. Prenatal Diagnosis—methods. QZ 50 P9235]
RG628.3.P74P73 1992
616'.042—dc20
DNLM/DLC
for Library of Congress 92–25339
CIP

The text of this book is printed on acid-free paper.

CONTENTS

CONTRIBUTORS

Reproductive Genetics Institute and Illinois Masonic Medical Center
Chicago, Illinois 60657

Jeanine Cieslak [49]

Paul De Sutter [93]

Andrey Dyban [93]

Norman Ginsberg [37]

Anver M. Kuliev [ix, 1, 5, 15, 19, 129, 139, 143]

Aaron Lifchez [37]

Svetlana Rechitsky [69]

Charles M. Strom [69]

Yury Verlinsky [ix, 1, 19, 49, 93, 129, 143]

The numbers in brackets are the opening page numbers of the contributors' articles.

PREFACE

Prevention of genetic disease currently requires prenatal diagnosis and selective abortion, which is a major limitation of the present technology available. This book introduces a new approach for the avoidance of congenital disease either through selection of unaffected gametes prior to fertilization or through selection of unaffected preembryos before implantation. This provides a very valuable option for genetically disadvantaged couples to avoid the birth of an affected child without the need for abortion. The book describes the original experience in the field of preimplantation genetic diagnosis, reviews the present knowledge in this exciting area, and addresses existing problems to be solved in the next few years. It puts together the advances in different areas of basic and applied research in IVF, embryology, micromanipulation and biopsy, DNA analysis of gametes and preembryos, and cytogenetic studies in preimplantation development relevant to preimplantation genetic diagnosis.

Preimplantation diagnosis is described in the framework of existing approaches for prevention of congenital disorders as natural evolution of the genetic technology into more ethically acceptable preventive measures. Although more research is needed before preimplantation genetic diagnosis can be widely applied in clinical practice, organizational aspects and possible indications for preimplantation genetic diagnosis are discussed. The most comprehensive description, however, is given to the existing approaches and practical techniques for oocyte and preembryo sampling, and to the methods for DNA and cytogenetic analysis in preimplantation development.

To make it possible to implement preimplantation diagnosis in the framework of IVF clinics, a detailed description of sampling techniques is extensively illustrated in Chapter 2. The chapter also contains a guide for preparation of the required media and a complete list of required materials and reagents.

The chapter on DNA analysis of polar bodies and preembryos contains a comprehensive guide for polymerase chain reaction (PCR) in single cells based on the long-standing original experience in the field. The list of primers and allele-specific oligonucleotides used for preimplantation diagnosis of different genetic diseases and a detailed description of reaction conditions for each primer and allele-specific oligonucleotide may be of great value in implementing the methods for preconception and preimplantation genetic diagnosis.

In view of the considerable contribution of chromosomal abnormalities in the early embryonic loss, and the importance of preimplantation diagnosis of chromosomal disorders, one of the chapters is devoted to the progress in cytogenetic analysis in preimplantation development. It contains a review of the current knowledge in the field, a comprehensive description of available techniques for making chromosomal preparations in preimplantation development, and also new information, based on the original work designed at the cytogenetic analysis of the first and second polar bodies.

In most of the chapters particular emphasis is placed on the existing problems and areas for future research. As preimplantation diagnosis raises important ethical issues, these issues are also briefly discussed. However, the book does not intend to completely cover this subject or other aspects of assisted procreation. On the contrary, laboratory aspects of preimplantation genetic diagnosis are described in more detail, with presentation of the original data, and are supported by lists of equipment and reagents needed for realization of each technique involved.

Finally, as preimplantation genetic diagnosis is a multidisciplinary approach, requiring an involvement of a team including obstetricians, fertility specialists, embryologists, geneticists, molecular biologists, and cytogeneticists, the book may be useful for a wide range of medical and biomedical personnel involved in assisted reproduction, genetics services, and maternal and child health care.

We thank Georg Wolf, Dimitry Dozortzev, and Susie Shore for their help in preparation of the manuscript.

Yury Verlinsky
Anver M. Kuliev

CHAPTER 1

Introduction

Yury Verlinsky and Anver M. Kuliev

The incidence of severe congenital and genetic disorders that can cause early death or lifelong chronic disease ranges from 15 to 45 per 1,000 live births; this includes congenital malformations (8 to 5 per 1,000), chromosomal anomalies (2 to 5 per 1,000) and Mendelian disorders (4 to 7 per 1,000) (Table I). The contribution of genetic as compared to nongenetic conditions in hospital admissions and the frequency of genetic disorders in some North American populations are presented in Table II.

The development of new methods for diagnosis of genetic disease in the early stages of development of the human zygote and embryo (before implantation) is particularly needed for couples having high recurrent risk for offspring with inherited diseases. In most of these cases the risk of having an affected child is as high as 25% in each pregnancy for recessively inherited and X-linked disorders, or as high as 50% in dominantly inherited disorders.

Preimplantation genetic diagnosis (PGD) will make it possible to overcome the most sensitive problem in the management of genetic disease—the problem of abortion, which, because it is not acceptable for some populations or ethnic groups, gives rise to negative reaction to preventive genetic programs. Therefore, earlier approaches to intervention provide a wider range of options for genetically disadvantaged people and may make medical genetics services more ethically acceptable.

The deliberations of the First International Symposium on Preimplantation Genetics (Verlinsky and Kuliev, 1991), have shown that the methods for detecting most genetic conditions after implantation could be applied, in principle, to gametes and preembryos. However, it is obvious that much research is still needed to adapt DNA methods, and cytogenetic and biochemical methods to PGD, particularly with respect to safety and diagnostic accuracy. These methods could be expected to be

Table I Estimated Frequency of Congenital Disorders[1]

Type of disorder	All disorders (incidence per 1,000 births)	Severe disorders (incidence per 1,000 births)
Congenital malformations	17–30	8–15
Chromosomal aberrations	4–9	2–5
Mendelian disorders	4–7	4–7
Hemoglobinopathies	0–16	0–16
Total	25–62	14–43

[1]From WHO, 1985

widely applied, first of all, for in vitro fertilization (IVF) patients, using the same criteria for identification of individuals and couples at genetic risk as for prenatal diagnosis.

The development of PGD seems a natural step in the evolution of genetic disease prevention technology from the stage when there was neither treatment nor genetic counseling and prenatal diagnosis, to the stage when all options including PGD are available (Kuliev and Modell, 1991). The availability of PGD could improve

Table II Frequency (%) of Genetic Disorders in Some North American Populations[1]

	In Hospital Admissions		In General Population
Type of Disorder	Pediatric	Adult	Total births
Genetic			
Chromosomal	0.4	0	0.18
Single Gene	5.5	1.5	0.36
Multifactorial	14.2	12.0	4.64
Congenital Malformations	23.0	0	3.22[2]
Multifactorial and Congenital together	35.7	—	—
"Familial"	11.2	—	0.12
Nongenetic	47.2	86.5	
Sample size (n)	30,597	3,298	1,169,873

[1]From Scriver, 1992.
[2]Congenital anomalies without identifiable genetic cause

specialized genetics services and related clinical practices, as it provides an option for those couples who cannot accept abortion as an obligatory step in the presently used control measures for avoiding a serious inherited disease. For example, when treatment and information on recurrence risk were introduced, many couples either refrained from reproduction or terminated their pregnancies, so that their family size decreased to less than that half of the population norm. With the introduction of community-based screening and prenatal diagnosis, the average family size of the couples at risk may be returned to nearly normal level, but at the cost of abortion of affected fetuses (Modell and Kuliev, 1991).

The expected impact of PGD on the existing policies for prevention of genetic disease is not only to allow the achievement of normal reproductive potential, but also to eliminate the need of terminating 25% of wanted pregnancies, as in case of prenatal diagnosis of autosomal recessive disease.

References

Kuliev AM, Modell B (1991): Ethical issues in the control of genetic diseases. In Verlinsky Y, Kuliev AM (eds): "Preimplantation Genetics." New York: Plenum Press, pp. 139–145.

Modell B, Kuliev AM (1991): Services for thalassemia as a model for cost–benefit analysis of genetics services. J Inher Metab Dis 14:640–651.

Scriver C (1992): Genetic disease: Effects on human health in Genetic services delivery: International Perspective. In Kuliev AM, Paul N, Penchassadeh V, Greendale K (eds): Birth Defects: Original Article Series, Vol 28, issue 3. New York: March of Dimes.

Verlinsky Y, Kuliev AM (eds) (1991): "Preimplantation Genetics." New York: Plenum Press.

WHO (1985): "Community approaches to the control of hereditary diseases." Report of a WHO Advisory Group; unpublished WHO document. HDP/WG/85.10. (May be obtained free of charge from The Hereditary Diseases Programme, WHO, Geneva, Switzerland).

CHAPTER 2

Approaches to Prevention of Genetic Diseases: The Place of Preimplantation Genetic Diagnosis in Prevention and Control of Congenital Disorders

Anver M. Kuliev

The main objective in the management of genetic disorders, as in other diseases, must be prevention where possible, and treatment where not. Unfortunately, prevention is usually impossible since many mutations have been established for generations, and even though we can try to prevent some increases in mutation rate, we cannot reverse the mutations that have occurred in the past (WHO, 1986). Treatment for most genetic disorders is also impossible at present (Hayes et al., 1985), and is unlikely ever to be effective in the large proportion of disorders, including chromosomal abnormalities and those severe genetic conditions in which pathological changes are already well established at birth. Even when treatment is effective, it is often lifelong and expensive, with the affected families needing intensive social and psychological support to cope with chronic disability and the danger of premature death, and to tolerate inconvenient and boring management regimens.

Since prevention can have little effect on most genetic disorders in the immediate future, and because so few respond to treatment, the only alternative in their management is avoidance, by diagnosis and carrier detection, thus making it possible to avoid the conception, implantation, or birth of affected children. This increases the chances of providing adequate medical and other services to survivors. Table I. presents methods of avoiding congenital disease for those at genetic risk.

Among the approaches for prevention of genetic disease is genetic counselling,

Table I Ways for Carriers to Avoid Having Children With Inherited Disease[1]

Time of Discovering Risk	Possible Action
Before marriage (uncommon)	1. Remain single (uncommon)
	2. Avoid selecting another carrier as partner (very uncommon)
	3. Select a partner in the usual way (the most common choice)
After marriage (more common)	4. Remain childless (common only for severe disease when PND impossible)
	5. "Take the chance" (common for less severe diseases)
	6. Use PND (very common)
	7. Use AID or other form of "assisted reproduction" (very uncommon)
	8. Use PGD (to be evaluated)
	9. Separate and find another partner (very uncommon)
After birth of an affected child (most common)	Options 4-8 above for further reproduction, plus:
	10. Accept infant and treatment (usual)
	11. Accept infant, but reject treatment (sometimes)
	12. Reject infant (can happen)

PND, prenatal diagnosis; AID, artificial insemination by donor; PGD, preimplantation genetic diagnosis. [1]Modified from RCP, 1989 and Kuliev, Modell, 1990.

which includes the provision of accurate information on genetic risk, and which is an integral and obligatory component of any attempts to manage genetic diseases. It is particularly important in screening programs, prenatal diagnosis, and preimplantation genetic diagnosis (PGD), since it enables people to use genetic information to avoid the risk of a serious congenital disease.

Before prenatal and preimplantation diagnosis was possible, the main effect of genetic counselling on the incidence of genetic disorders was the prevention of transmission by modifying the reproductive behavior of those who were found to be carriers, or who were at risk of being carriers. The approach was based mainly on the diagnosis of the presenting affected child, i.e., was "retrospective" and oriented towards avoiding recurrence. However, its effectiveness was limited by many factors. In most developed countries the average family size is very small so the chance of a second affected child is already low; in addition, most congenital diseases are sporadic, and therefore would escape being a target of retrospective counselling. Thus, diagnosis of a dominant disorder in potential parents could lead them to avoid having children. However, in practice only a minority of those who know they might convey such disorders request advice. Further, many dominant disorders arise from new mutations in infants born to normal parents, and are therefore unpredictable.

In X-linked disorders, because of the high incidence of new mutations, family history may not be of help in estimating the risk of recurrence. Duchenne's muscular dystrophy (DMD) is one such disorder; it is never transmitted through affected males owing to disability and early death. In hemophilia, another X-linked disorder, even if patients are well informed, few choose to remain childless.

In the case of recessive disorders, because both parents are carriers, only a quarter of couples would have an affected first child, and only a quarter of these would produce a second affected child. Accordingly, genetic counselling alone is hardly likely to reduce the number of affected children significantly, although a greater degree of reduction would be possible in large families.

There is also little prospect that genetic counselling would have an appreciable effect on chromosomal diseases other than translocations, which are rare. The same is true for most congenital malformations, where the true risk of recurrence is usually unknown.

Clearly, voluntary childlessness as a result of genetic counselling, even if it were acceptable, is largely ineffective in reducing the incidence of genetic disorders, and in the future is unlikely to make any substantial impact on most diseases, unless advice based on the probability of being a carrier is replaced by definitive carrier diagnosis, as shown below.

Because every individual, couple, or even community may be at some genetic risk, the development of approaches for the identification of groups at risk is one of the key components in preventing genetic disease. Experience shows that some periods in an individual's life are particularly relevant for screening purposes, such as after birth, before marriage, or during pregnancy. These are times when possible genetic risks can be assessed. Analysis of experience in this field makes it possible to outline the existing problems in genetic screening.

Well-known examples of identification of groups at risk are those for phenylketonuria (PKU) and congenital hypothyroidism. The screening techniques for these have spread almost worldwide, although population coverage is poor in many areas. In some populations neonatal screening is being extended to sickle-cell disease (as in Cuba, and some areas of France, the United Kingdom, and the United States), and glucose-6-phosphate dehydrogenase (G6PD) deficiency (as in Singapore and some parts of Southern Europe). Some congenital malformations may also be diagnosed routinely in newborns, when early corrective treatment is possible. An example of this is early diagnosis of congenital dislocation of the hip, as demonstrated in Hungary (Czeizel and Tusnady, 1984). In a few countries, neonatal screening is also practiced for galactosemia and a few other inborn errors of metabolism, or for karyotyping.

There is a great need for the development of accurate neonatal screening tests for most common genetic diseases, with cystic fibrosis (CF) being one of the first candidates. Here, the aim is not only to attempt to improve the prognosis, but also to avoid the birth of another affected child. The immunoreactive trypsin test on dried blood spots, useful for research purposes in the past, is unacceptable in practice because of high rates of false positives and false negatives; however, the recently introduced DNA method appears to be reliable and is being incorporated into existing genetic programs, such as maternal serum alpha-fetoprotein (MSAFP) screening and prenatal diagnosis. Neonatal screening for alpha-1-antitrypsin deficiency has been undertaken in an attempt to avoid the risk of juvenile cirrhosis and emphysema in some homozygotes (McNeil et al., 1988).

Among the general problems in neonatal screening is inadequate coverage of the population. Even in Europe, coverage is not complete for any of the conditions mentioned (Kuliev and Modell, 1987); for example, only about a third of babies born in Europe are tested for congenital hypothyroidism, despite the high effectiveness and low cost of the procedure. Nevertheless, over a thousand affected infants are diagnosed and treated annually. With neonatal PKU screening, there appear to be no reliable measures for avoiding the development of mental retardation and congenital malformations in the offspring of affected females, so that damage may only be postponed for one generation. Therefore, as experience is gained, carriers of PKU may become candidates for prenatal or preimplantation, rather than neonatal, diagnosis, according to the choice of the couples concerned.

Finally, perhaps the most difficult problem in neonatal screening is to provide counselling for everyone involved, and to ensure monitoring of the results. At present, information for parents prior to testing has been rather neglected, although this is of particular importance in those disorders where both carriers and affected infants are detected, as in the case of sickle cell disease. The lack of appropriate information for participants of screening programs may also lead to serious ethical and social problems in conditions where the screening tests are not reliable, or in conditions which have low predictability.

A variety of techniques are available for genetic screening before and during pregnancy. These include ultrasound scanning in pregnancy, maternal serum screening for congenital malformations and chromosomal diseases, cytogenetic prenatal monitoring in connection with maternal age, premarital carrier detection in particular ethnic groups, and carrier screening in pregnancy for common genetic disorders. As excellent reviews on these techniques are available, only some technical and social aspects, relevant for prenatal and preimplantation diagnosis, are presented below.

In spite of the fact that there are still no controlled follow-up studies on its safety, ultrasound examination during pregnancy has become a basic routine procedure worldwide. The use of this procedure for obstetric purposes provides considerable potential for genetic screening, which might be even more fully utilized. For example, about 80% of fetuses destined to abort spontaneously could be identified by ultrasound 2 to 4 weeks before abortion occurred. Because in about half of the cases abortion stems from chromosomal abnormalities, this risk might be identified by routine ultrasound scanning in the first trimester, and unnecessary emergency problems could be avoided. When such screening cannot be provided for the community at large, it should at least be available for women over 35 years of age, as they face more than a 20% risk of a nonviable pregnancy (Stein et al., 1980).

Another problem with ultrasound scanning is the provision of a high-standard fetal-anomaly screening for every woman in the second and/or third trimester of pregnancy. Confining use of this technique to particular risk groups is inappropriate, because most congenital malformations occur without any prior indication of risk. On the other hand, widespread usage is handicapped by the lack of established standards for service organization and diagnosis, and of any agreed upon system for monitoring results. It may be possible to monitor the outcome of routine ultrasound scanning by concurrently observing changes in the incidence of congenital malformations among live-born infants, and the outcome of terminations of pregnancy for fetal abnormalities. Long-standing monitoring systems for birth defects could be used for the above purposes. Recent experience in the use of ultrasound scanning in the second and third trimesters of pregnancy opens new possibilities both for identifying groups at risk from chromosome-linked diseases, and also for improving neonatal surgical management of congenital malformations, such as congenital heart or renal disease.

Screening of maternal serum alpha-fetoprotein (MSAFP) has reduced the incidence of neural tube defects (NTDs) in the United Kingdom by at least 50% (Cuckle et al., 1989). A similar effect was demonstrated in Hungary, where the Hungarian Center for Congenital Anomaly Control has shown a decrease of up to 62% in the incidence of NTDs (Czeizel, 1988). However, the application of MSAFP screening was very limited, even in European countries, until it was shown to be useful for detecting pregnancies where there was a risk of chromosomal disease (Merkatz et al., 1984; Cuckle et al., 1987). Although such programs were just recently at the research stage, their potential importance for the avoidance of such diseases at the community level is already clear. The observation that the predictive power of MSAFP screening for chromosomal disorders can be greatly increased when it is combined with the screening of levels of other maternal serum factors, such as a low level of unconjugated estriol and a high level of chorionic gonadotropin (Bogart et al., 1987; Canick et al., 1988), has greatly increased the extent of routine screening of maternal serum. Searches for additional maternal serum factors of value in the identification of genetic risk, and studies of the feasibility of maternal serum screening in the first trimester of pregnancy are now under way to improve the effectiveness of maternal serum screening (Bogart et al., 1989; Bogart and Jones, 1991; Crandal et al., 1991; Kratzer et al., 1991, Brambati et al., 1992).

Advanced maternal age is strongly linked to the frequency of chromosomal disorders, and provides an opportunity for the identification of pregnancies at risk. The risk can be reduced by controlling reproduction in the advanced maternal age group, either through contraception or through induced abortion if the contraception policy fails. For example, about 50% of recognized pregnancies are aborted in Eastern European countries, these being predominantly among older women, whereas in

Western Europe induced abortions are commoner among young women wishing to postpone childbearing. The proportion of pregnancies at risk for chromosomal disorders differs greatly in each country according to maternal age distribution (Modell et al., 1991).

The other approach to identify those at risk for producing a genetically affected fetus is premarital screening. Although it has not been popular in most populations, when accepted, this approach showed a great impact on the prevention of genetic disease at the community level. The best example of this is Cyprus, where the premarital detection of carriers has been used to identify couples at risk for thalassemias (Angastiniotis et al., 1986). As all marriages there are registered in church, all persons are asked for a certificate stating that they have had heterozygote screening and counselling before they can be married. If both partners appear to be carriers of thalassemia genes, they would subsequently be able to avoid the disease through fetal diagnosis and selective abortion. Because the screening test is simple and accurate, the program has resulted in the complete elimination of new cases of this disease in the area.

Carrier detection before and during pregnancy is widely used in the identification of groups at risk for Tay-Sach's disease, sickle-cell disease, and thalassemias. For example, about 4% of people of Eastern European Jewish extraction are heterozygous for Tay-Sach's disease and can be identified by measuring the plasma level of the enzyme hexosaminidase A. Population screening for Tay-Sach's disease among groups at risk has been established in the United States, Canada, and Israel, and is being developed in the United Kingdom. Similar screening programs could be considered appropriate in other areas where the proportion of people of Jewish extraction is significant. It appears that in the United States the program has been highly effective, leading to a decrease of over a 90% in the birth incidence of this disease (Kaback, 1991). Population screening in pregnancy for the sickle-cell trait is practiced in Cuba and has proved effective in the identification of couples at risk and in reducing the number of newborns with the disease by about 30% (Heredero et al., 1991).

Screening in pregnancy to identify couples at risk for thalassemias has become a routine practice in many areas of the world. For example, in the European region as a whole, the birthrate of infants with thalassemia major is at least 0.18 per 1000, and it is endemic in the south of the region (WHO, 1987). Since the thalassemia trait causes a characteristic microcytic blood picture, thalassemia carriers can be detected easily and cheaply by means of automated equipment, followed by hemoglobin A_2 estimation. The need to establish a screening program may be estimated from the proportion in the population of the particular ethnic groups at risk for thalassemias, or from the proportion of births in these groups. When combined with prenatal diagnosis, these programs appeared to be highly effective, as can be seen from the recent evaluation of ongoing programs in Europe and Mediterranean countries (Modell and Kuliev, 1991).

The rapid development of DNA methods provides the possibility of developing carrier tests for certain common inherited diseases, such as CF as mentioned previously.

With the implementation of prenatal diagnosis and PGD, it becomes possible to replace childlessness as the only choice for a couple, with the chance of having a healthy child. In fact, the primary objective of prenatal and preimplantation diagnosis is not to eliminate the affected gamete, embryo, or child, but to ensure delivery of the desired number of healthy ones. Implementation of prenatal diagnosis has made preventive programs highly effective. For example, although it is only applicable to those who accept fetal death as an alternative to a crippled childhood, experience has shown that in most communities the majority of women with a high or even a low risk of producing a seriously affected child readily accept fetal diagnosis. With recent improvements in sampling techniques and DNA methods, the acceptance rate of fetal diagnosis has increased considerably, as can be seen from the experience of leading prenatal diagnosis centers (Table II) (Galjaard, 1991). The demand for fetal diagnosis is enormous, as can be demonstrated by the number of pregnancies among women of advanced maternal age and the number of common avoidable genetic disorders (Modell, et al., 1991). Nevertheless, there are limitations in the application of fetal diagnosis; these are due to the fact that biochemical defects and the molecular (DNA) etiology are known only for about 15% of genetic disorders (McKusick, 1990; Gindilis, 1991). Another limitation of this type of diagnosis is the unavailability of screening tests for some conditions which could be diagnosed in the fetus. For example, most children with chromosomal diseases are born because the pregnancies at risk are not identified, and thus they are not referred for prenatal diagnosis.

Any wider application of fetal diagnosis will also depend on considerations of the

Table II Increase in Referral for Prenatal Diagnosis[1,2]

	Number of pregnant women investigated							
Diagnostic method	1980	1981	1982	1984	1985	1986	1987	1989
Amniocentesis	900	1062	1220	1471	1679	1767	1641	1239
Transcervical CVS	—	—	—	205	319	490	491	90
Transabdominal CVS	—	—	—	—	—	—	216	947
Ultrasound examination for fetal anomaly	dozens	many dozens	few hundreds	570	776	873	1020	1634

[1]Rotterdam, The Netherlands (1970-1990) (Galjaard, 1991)
[2]1970: start of programme; 1976: 6% of women > 38 years; 1980: 20% of women > 38 years; 1990: 60% of women > 36 years

short-term and long-term risks of obstetric procedures such as amniocentesis, fetal blood sampling, and chorionic villus sampling (CVS). Well-designed research programs carried out to evaluate the obstetric risk of CVS did not indicate an excessive rate of fetal loss (Canadian Collaborative CVS-Amniocentesis Clinical Trial Group 1989; USNICHD, 1990). A recent discussion on this issue has demonstrated the importance of carrying out these procedures in specialized centers to avoid a possible risk from CVS testing in the first trimester of pregnancy (Mahoney, 1991; Fifth et al., 1991; Hsiem et al., 1991; Mastroiacovo and Cavalcanti, 1991; Jackson et al., 1991; Monni et al, 1991; Miny et al, 1991). A wider application of prenatal diagnosis will also strongly depend upon the accuracy of laboratory diagnosis (Ledbetter et al., 1992). There is a need to improve existing cytogenetic, biochemical, and DNA methods which could also be applicable for PGD. These need to be made more reliable and simpler, and accurate tests for conditions which are not diagnosable at present are also required.

The major limitation of prenatal diagnosis, as mentioned, is that affected fetuses have to be aborted. The development of approaches for PGD may help to solve this problem by making the measures for preventing genetic diseases more ethically acceptable, since it removes abortion as an obligatory step in the program (Verlinsky and Kuliev, 1991). Thus an even more important point is that PGD provides wider options for individuals and couples at risk of bearing an abnormal fetus, as those who cannot accept prenatal diagnosis and abortion may choose gamete or preembryo diagnosis so that no pregnancy has to be selectively interrupted. Therefore, the elimination of an affected fetus, a major "cost" for having an unaffected child in the currently available preventive programs, is avoided by PGD, which extends the options for couples, who may reproduce without the need for interrupting a wanted pregnancy following prenatal diagnosis.

The experience of introduction of PGD, described in Chapters 4 and 7, will show that it seems acceptable, at least for in vitro fertilization (IVF) couples at high risk for conceiving a child with an inherited disease.

References

Angastiniotis MA, Kyriakidou S, Hadjiminas M (1986): How thalassaemia was controlled in Cyprus. World Health Forum 7:291–297.

Bogart MH, Golbus MS, Sorg ND, Jones OW (1989): Human chorionic gonadotropin levels in pregnancies with aneuploid fetuses. Prenat Diagn 9:379–384.

Bogart MH, Pandian MR, Jones OW (1987): Abnormal chorionic gonadotropin levels in pregnancies with fetal chromosome abnormalities. Prenat Diagn 7:623–630.

Bogart MH, Jones OW (1991): Prenatal screening for fetal Down's syndrome. Prenat Diagn 11:763–765.

Brambati B, Macintosh MCM, Teisner B, McGuiness S, Skrimanker K, Lanzami H, bonachi A, Tului L, grudzinskas JG (1992): Low maternal serum level of Pregnancy-associated plasma protein A(PAPP-A) in the first trimester in association with abnormal fetal karyotype. Brit J Obstet Gynecol (in press).

Canadian Collaborative CVS–Amniocentesis Clinical Trial Group (1989): Multicentre randomised clinical trial of chorion villus sampling and amniocentesis. Lancet 1:1–6.

Canick JA, Knight GJ, Palomaki GE, Haddow JE, Cuckle HS, Wald NJ (1988): Low-second trimester maternal serum unconjugated oestriol in pregnancies with Down's syndrome. Br J Obstet Gynaecol 95:330–333.

Crandal BF, Golbus MS, Goldberg JD, Matsumoto M (1991): First-trimester maternal serum unconjugated oestriol and alpha-fetoprotein in fetal Down's syndrome. Prenat Diagn 11:377–380.

Cuckle HS, Wald NJ, Cuckle PM (1989): Antenatal diagnosis of neural tube defects in England and Wales. Prenat Diagn 9:393–400.

Cuckle HS, Wald NJ, Thompson SG (1987): Estimating a woman's risk of having a pregnancy associated with Down's syndrome using her age and serum alpha-fetoprotein level. Br J Obstet Gynecol 94:387–402.

Czeizel A, Tusnady G (1984): "Aetiological studies of isolated congenital anomalies in Hungary". Budapest: Akadémiai Kiadó.

Czeizel A (1988): Neural tube defects. JAMA 259:3562

Fifth HV, Boyd PA, Chamberlain P, MacKenzie IZ, Lindenbaum RH, Huson SM (1991): Severe limb abnormalities after chorion villus sampling at 56–66 days' gestation. Lancet 337:782–783.

Galjaard H (1991): Antenatal diagnosis of fetal abnormalities. In Drife JO, Donnai D (eds): "Antenatal Diagnosis of Fetal Abnormalities." London: Springer-Verlag.

Gindilis V (1991): Human Genome Encyclopedia. Moscow: VINITI (in Russian).

Hayes A, Costa T, Scriver C, Childs B (1985): The effect of Mendelian disease on human health. II. Response to treatment. Am J Med Genet 21:243–255.

Heredero L, Granda H, Rodriguez L, Menendez F, Lantigua A, Oliva JA, Barrios B, Guerra D (1991): Implementation of hereditary disease programme in Cuba. Proceedings of the 8th International Congress of Human Genetics. Am J Hum Genet (Suppl) 49 , 4:321.

Hsiem FJ, Chen D, Tseng LH, Lee CN, Ko TM, Chuange SM, Chen HY (1991): Limb reduction defects and chorionic villus sampling. Lancet 337:1091–1092.

Jackson LG, Wapner RJ, Brambati B (1991): Limb abnormalities and chorionic villus sampling. Lancet 337:1091.

Kaback M, Lim-Steele J, Johnson D, Dabholkar D, Brown D, Levy N, Zeiger K (1991): The control of Tay-Sach's (TSD): A one generation assessment. Proceedings of the 8th International Congress of Human Genetics. Am J Hum Genet (Suppl) 49, 4:42.

Kratzer PG, Golbus MS, Monroe SE, Finkelstein DE, Taylor RN (1991): First-trimester aneuploidy screening using serum human chorionic gonadotropin (HCG), free hCG, and progesterone. Prenat Diagn 11:751–765.

Kuliev AM, Modell B (1991): Ethical issues in the control of genetic diseases. In Verlinsky Y, Kuliev AM (eds): "Preimplantation Genetics." New York: Plenum Press, pp. 233–244.

Kuliev AM, Modell B (1990): Problems in the control of genetic disorders. Biomed Sci 1:3–17.

Kuliev AM, Modell B (1987): "Community Genetics Services in Europe." Available from the Maternal and Child Health Unit, WHO Regional Office for Europe, 8 Scherfigsvej, DK-2100 Copenhagen, Denmark.

Ledbetter DH, Zachary JM, Simpson JL, Golbus MS, Pergament E, Jackson L, Mahoney MJ, Desnick RJ, Schulman J, Copeland KL, Verlinsky Y, Yang-Feng T, Schonberg SA, Babu A, Tharapel A, Dorfmann A, Lubs HA, Rhoads GG, Fowler SE, de la Cruz F (1992): Cytogenetic results from the U.S. collaborative study on CVS: High diagnostic accuracy in over 11,000 cases. Prenat Diagn 12: 317–345.

Mahoney MJ, for the USNICHD Collaborative CVS Study Group (1991): Limb abnormalities and chorion villus sampling. Lancet 337:1422–1423.

Mastroiacovo P, Cavalcanti DP (1991): Limb reduction defects and chorion villus sampling. Lancet 337:1091.

McKusick V (1990): "Mendelian Inheritance in Man," 9th Ed. Baltimore, MD: Johns Hopkins University Press.

McNeil TF, Sveger T, Thelin T (1988): Psychosocial aspects of screening for somatic risk: the Swedish α-1-antitrypsin experience. Thorax 43:505–507.

Merkatz IR, Nitowsky HM, Macri JN, Johnson WE (1984): An association between low maternal serum alpha-fetoprotein and fetal chromosome abnormalities. Am J Obstet Gynecol 148:886–891.

Miny P, Holzgreve W, Horst J, Lenz W (1991): Limb abnormalities and chorionic villus sampling. Lancet 337:1422–1423.

Modell B, Kuliev A (1991): Services for thalassaemia as a model for cost-benefit analysis of genetics services. J Inher Metab Dis 14:640–651.

Modell B, Kuliev A, Wagner M (1991): "Community Genetic Services in Europe." WHO Regional Publications. European Series No. 38. Available from the WHO Regional Office for Europe, 8 Scherfigsuej, DK-2100 Copenhagen, Denmark.

Monni G, Ibra RM, Lai R, Olla G, Cao A (1991): Limb reduction defects and chorion villus sampling. Lancet 337:1091.

Royal College of Physicians (RCP) (1989): "Prenatal Diagnosis and Genetic Screening." Community and service implications report of the Royal College of Physicians, Royal College of Physicians. London, UK.

Stein Z, Kline J, Susser E, Shrout P, Warburton D, Susser M (1980): Maternal age and spontaneous abortion. In Hook EB, Porter IH (eds): "Human Embryonic and Fetal Death." New York: Academic Press. pp. 107–127.

USNICHD Collaborative CVS Study Group (1990): Transcervical and transabdominal chorionic villus sampling are comparably safe procedures for first trimester prenatal diagnosis: Preliminary analysis. Am J Hum Genet 47:A278 (abstract).

Verlinsky Y, Kuliev AM (eds) (1991): "Preimplantation Genetics." New York: Plenum Press.

WHO (1986) Report of a Task Group: Prevention of avoidable mutational disease. Bull World Health Org 64:205–216.

WHO (1987): The haemoglobinopathies in Europe. Report of two meetings of the WHO European/Mediterranean Working Group on Haemoglobinopathies. IPC/MCH 110, WHO Regional Office for Europe. Available from the Maternal and Child Health Unit, WHO Regional Office for Europe, 8 Scherfigsvej, DK–2100, Copenhagen, Denmark.

CHAPTER 3

Indications for and Organization of Preimplantation Genetic Diagnosis

Anver M. Kuliev

Indications for preimplantation genetic diagnosis (PGD) could be, in principle, the same as for prenatal diagnosis, but at the moment PGD is justified only for high risk pregnancies. For example, the risk for neural tube defects, one of major indications for amniocentesis, is indeed not the case for PGD. Maternal age, the other major indication for prenatal diagnosis, is not expected to be the indication for such early diagnosis either, not only because PGD of chromosomal diseases has not yet been worked out to the extent of practical application, but because advanced maternal age could be considered as an obstetric contraindication of PGD (Milunsky, 1991). Among the other obstetric and genetic contraindications of PGD, Milunsky listed the following: habitual abortions; a seriously adverse obstetric history including recurrent premature ruptured membranes and early and severe preeclamptic toxemia, anatomical uterine abnormalities; persistent or serious pregnancy-induced hypertension; insulin-dependent diabetes; maternal epilepsy, maternal cystic fibrosis (CF), sickle-cell disease, myotonic muscular dystrophy, or connective tissue disorders such as Marfan's or Ehlers-Danlos' syndrome.

Although the organizational aspects of PGD are not clear at the moment, since PGD seems to be an obvious extension of prenatal diagnosis and of in vitro fertilization (IVF), the same referral system could be used for prenatal diagnosis, so that couples who cannot accept terminating a pregnancy could be offered a genetic diagnosis before implantation. Another approach to reaching the couples in need of PGD is to offer genetic screening for the most prevalent congenital conditions within the IVF or prenatal diagnosis programs. Primary target diseases would be CF in

Caucasian populations, hemoglobinopathies in Mediterranean groups, or Tay-Sach's disease in Jewish communities.

Experience with wide-scale screening for hemoglobinopathies and CF is already available, and shows the possible scope of PGD for these conditions.

One of the best examples of carrier screening for hemoglobinopathies has been developed in Sardinia (Cao et al., 1990), and is carried out voluntarily at child-bearing age with or without ongoing pregnancy. The testing of 167,000 people resulted in the identification of 35,500 β-thalassemia carriers and 1,544 couples at risk. By adding to this figure the number of known couples at risk (those having affected children in the family), the total number of identified couples at risk (2,356) approached 87% of the total predicted on the basis of carrier rate in the population, which is 1 out of 8 individuals (1 out of 60 couples). After the introduction of first-trimester fetal diagnosis about 99% of counseled couples accepted prenatal diagnosis, but 0.7% of those in whom an affected fetus was diagnosed still decided to continue pregnancy because they were against interrupting a pregnancy, This group would be candidates for PGD.

To evaluate the degree of acceptability of PGD, a specially designed study was organized in this population by inviting couples with a prior experience of selective abortion following prenatal diagnosis to join an experimental PGD program. Of the interviewed couples, 75% signed the waiting list for PGD, an unexpectedly high acceptance rate (Brambati and Formigli, 1991). Similar observations were made in the United Kingdom's thalassemia control program, where couples with prior experience of prenatal diagnosis were interviewed (B. Modell, personal communication).

Although the experience of carrier screening for CF is much smaller than that for hemoglobinopathies, the results are in accordance with the above. In London, of an interviewed community sample indicated their willingness to be tested (Watson et al., 1991). The introduction of CF screening confirmed this observation, as CF carrier testing was undertaken by 66% of patients in general practices, and 87% of patients in family planning clinics (R. Williamson, personal communication).

The introduction of prenatal diagnosis of CF has changed the reproductive behavior of couples at risk of conceiving an affected child. For example, in the California study (Kaback et al., 1984) 62% of couples had undergone surgical sterilization following the birth of a CF child in the family. In the Paris study, 75% of the couples with a CF child had no subsequent pregnancy (Boué et al., 1991). However, the majority of these couples had two or more successive pregnancies when prenatal diagnosis of CF became available. Boué et al., (1991) demonstrated that when the result of prenatal diagnosis was a normal fetus, 16.5% of couples had a further pregnancy after the birth of the normal infant. It can be predicted, that with the option for PGD the proportion of couples at risk who decide to remain childless will be lower, as even those who cannot accept selective abortion could achieve a desired family size. Reaching such families will depend on the availability of community screening programs which are not generally acceptable. Some guidelines used for performing CF screening in the United States can be derived from the statement of the NIH (Workshop on Population Screening for Cystic Fibrosis Gene, 1990) and the recommendations of the National Academy of Science (Committee on Inborn Errors of Metabolism, 1975). In European countries also there is no population screening policy yet, though specially designed pilot programs are under way, such as the previously mentioned pilot program initiated in the United Kingdom by the Cystic Fibrosis Research Trust.

Another approach for reaching couples in need of preimplantation genetic diagnosis for CF is implementation of CF screening in in vitro fertilization and prenatal diagnosis settings. For example, prenatal screening for CF was extended in patients undergoing chorionic villus sampling (CVS) or amniocentesis (Maddalena et al., 1991). Concurrent CF testing of their fetal sample was offered to 3,219 consecutive patients. The test was accepted by 43.5% of CVS patients and 19.7% of amniocentesis patients.

Our experience with the introduction of CF screening among CVS and IVF patients also suggests the acceptability of the test. The results of PGD for the couple identified in this study will be described in Chapter 7.

As experience in implementing prenatal diagnosis has already shown, it would be expected that initially PGD could be provided only in a few specialized centers for fetal medicine, since it is a multidisciplinary approach requiring the involvement of personnel highly specialized in areas such as obstetrics, ultrasonography, embryology, cytogenetics, clinical and molecular genetics. Such a team approach was instrumental in the development of CVS and fetal blood sampling and has led to the development of a new area in medical research—fetal medicine. The team approach in IVF and specialized genetics programs will serve as an appropriate basis for offering PGD within existing structures which provide genetics services.

The application of PGD will also depend on the cost, which is now too high to be afforded generally. However, with the progress both in IVF and in genetic analysis, the cost of PGD can be expected to decrease substantially. It is too early to consider the cost-effectiveness of this new option for avoiding genetic diseases, but the nonfinancial benefits involved are so great for the couples at high genetic risk, that the provision of PGD as a matter of choice may be justified.

References

Boué J, Muller F, Simon-Buoy B, Faure C, and Boué A (1991): Consequences of prenatal diagnosis of cystic fibrosis on the reproductive attitudes of parents of affected children. Prenat Diagn 11:209–214.

Brambati B, Formigli L (1991): Uterine lavage for preimplantation genetic diagnosis. In Verlinsky Y, Kuliev AM (eds): "Preimplantation Genetics." New York: Plenum Press, pp. 165–174.

Cao A, Rosatelli C, Leom GB, Tuveri T, Scalas MT, Monni O, Galanello R (1990): Antenatal diagnosis of ß-thalassemia in Sardinia. Ann N Y Acad Sci 612:215–225.

Committee on Inborn Errors of Metabolism (1975): Genetic screening: programs, principles and research. Washington, DC: National Academy of Sciences.

Kaback M, Ziplin D, Boyd P, Cantor R (1984): Attitude towards prenatal diagnosis of cystic fibrosis among parents of affected children. In Lawsons D (ed): "Cystic Fibrosis: Horizons." Chichester: John Wiley, pp 15–28.

Maddalena A, Bick DP, Black SH, Hansma DI, Cummings E, Jones SL, Fallon L, Headrick EG, Schulman JD (1991): Prenatal screening for cystic fibrosis (CF) in United States couples without a previously affected child. Proceedings of the 8th International Congress of Human Genetics. Am J Hum Genet Suppl 49, 4:329.

Milunsky A (1991): Ethical and selected medical aspects of preimplantation genetic diagnosis. In Verlinsky Y, Kuliev AM (eds): "Preimplantation Genetics." New York: Plenum Press, pp. 245–252.

Watson EK, Williamson R, Chapple J (1991): Attitudes to carrier screening for cystic fibrosis: a survey of health care professionals, relatives of sufferers and other members of the public. Br J General Pract 41:237–240.

Workshop on Population Screening for the Cystic Fibrosis Gene (1990): Statement from the National Institute of Health Workshop on Population Screening for the Cystic Fibrosis Gene. N Engl J Med 323:70–71.

CHAPTER 4

Approaches to Preimplantation Genetic Diagnosis

Yury Verlinsky and Anver M. Kuliev

Considering the perspectives on fetal diagnosis of genetic disease in 1984, the World Health Organization (WHO) stressed the relevance of developing earlier approaches for genetic analysis, with the possibility of diagnosing genetic disease before implantation (WHO, 1984; Kuliev et al., 1985). The following possibilities for preimplantation genetic diagnosis (PGD) were mentioned: genetic analysis of the first or second polar bodies, and embryo biopsy at the cleavage or blastocyst stage (WHO, 1984; McLaren, 1985; Kuliev et al., 1985). However, realization of some of these approaches become possible only after introduction of the polymerase chain reaction (PCR) (Saiki et al., 1985) and success in developing micromanipulation and embryo biopsy techniques.

Attempts at PGD were undertaken in mammalian embryos only about five years ago (Leonard et al., 1987; Monk et al., 1988; Monk and Handyside, 1988; Summers et al., 1988; Gordon and Gang, 1990). These demonstrated that material could be removed from mammalian preembryos and successfully analyzed without destroying the viability of the preembryo.

The first real possibilities for PGD of human genetic disease were demonstrated by Handyside et al. (1989) for X-linked diseases, and by Verlinsky et al. (1990) for autosomal recessive diseases. Children without detectable birth defects have been born following these procedures (Handyside et al., 1990), demonstrating that embryo biopsy can be performed safely in humans.

The above studies have also introduced the two main approaches for genetic diagnosis before implantation: (1) PGD based on biopsy of gametes; and (2) PGD based on preembryo biopsy. A review of the developments in preconception and

Table I Effect of Polar Body Removal on Fertilization and Cleavage[1]

	Cycles	Oocytes	Fractured or Atretic	Fertilized Monospermic	Dispermic	Total	Cleaved[2]
With PBR							
	10	121	29	54/92 59%	7/92 8%	61/92 66%	54/54 100%
Without PBR							
	40	266	30	151/236 64%	12/236 5%	163/236 69%	147/151 97%

[1]From Verlinsky, 1991.
[2]Triploid embryos not included.

preimplantation genetic diagnosis, and of existing problems in the possible application of these early approaches to clinical practice, are presented below.

Preconception Genetic Analysis

Biopsy of gametes opens an intriguing possibility for preconception diagnosis of inherited diseases, as genetic analysis of biopsied gamete material will make it feasible to select gametes containing unaffected alleles for fertilization and subse-

Table II Preimplantation Development Following Polar Body Removal and Blastomere Biopsy

Oocytes	PBR	Fertilized			PBR	Transfer	Cultured to blastocyst		
		2N	3N	Total	+BB		PBR only	PBR +BB	Total
Mature									
114	111	87	6	93	62	32	4	28[1]	32
Immature									
27	18	3	0	3	1	2	0	0	0
Total									
141	129	90	6	96	63	34	4	28	32

[1]Four blastomeres were frozen and transferred in subsequent cycles.

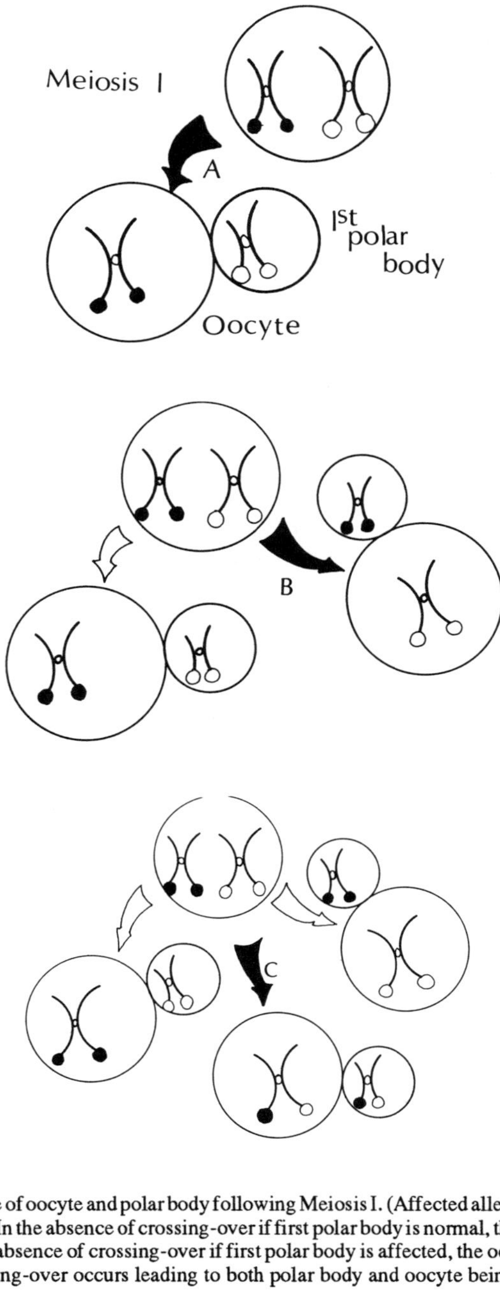

Figure 1 Genotype of oocyte and polar body following Meiosis I. (Affected alleles are shown as dark dots): **A.** In the absence of crossing-over if first polar body is normal, the oocyte is affected; **B.** In the absence of crossing-over if first polar body is affected, the oocyte will be normal. **C.** Crossing-over occurs leading to both polar body and oocyte being heterozygous.

Table III Clinical Trial of Preconception Diagnosis

	Disease				
	CF	HA	A1-AT	TSD	
Number of					Total
Couples	5	1	1	1	8
Cycles	7	5	5	3	20

CF = Cystic Fibrosis, HA = Hemophilia, A1-AT = α–1–antitrypsin deficiency, TSD = Tay-Sach's Disease

quent transfer. In this way, it is possible to avoid not only selective abortion of an affected fetus, but also fertilization involving affected gametes.

Although preconception genetic diagnosis could be achieved by genotyping either oocytes or sperm, the latter approach is not realistic at the present time. Despite extensive studies, claims to have successfully separated X and Y spermatozoa, in order to prevent X-linked disorders, have not been confirmed. Also, no method exists to retain the viability of sperm after analyzing its genotype, although PCR now permits the genotyping of individual human sperm (Li et al., 1988; 1991; Coutelle et al., 1989; Arnheim et al., 1990, 1991). The development of methods for culturing primary spermatocytes and spermatogonia followed by genetic analysis of mature spermatid may theoretically be possible, but this still remains a subject for future research.

The only approach for preconception diagnosis at present, therefore, seems to be the genotyping of oocytes, by micromanipulation and biopsy, with subsequent genetic analysis of biopsied material.

It is possible to obtain the genotype of an oocyte by direct analysis, but this analysis destroys the oocyte. To overcome this obstacle an approach has been developed to genotype the oocyte by removing the first polar body and performing genetic analysis of its DNA (Verlinsky et al., 1990). Figure 1 demonstrates the possible events following meiosis and how these affect prediction of a genotype of the oocyte. In the absence of crossing-over, the first polar body will be homozygous for the allele not contained in the oocyte and second polar body. If crossing-over occurs, the oocyte will be heterozygous and the eventual genotype of the oocyte cannot be predicted. The frequency of crossing-over will vary with the distance between the locus and the centromere. For telomeric genes the crossover frequency approaches 50%, while for genes close to the centromere the frequency may be close to zero.

Even with telomeric genes, 50% of the polar bodies will be homozygous, and half of these (25%) will be homozygous for the mutant allele indicating that the oocytes contain the normal allele and can be used for fertilization and transfer. Since preconception genetic diagnosis involves induction of superovulation, several folli-

Table IV Preconception Genetic Analysis[1]

	Genotype of the Oocytes After Polar Body Removal				
	Normal	Heterozygous	Affected	Failed PCR	Total
Cystic Fibrosis (delta F-508)	5	5	8	4	22
Hemophilia[2]	21	19	9	13	62
α-1-Antitrypsin[3] Deficiency	13	27	6	5	51
Tay-Sach's disease	3	2	2	3	10
Total	42	53	25	25	145

[1]The numbers show the number of polar bodies studied.
[2]Analysis of the HbaI polymorphism in amplified DNA. (The absence of XbaI site in this family, i.e., hybridization to probe 7.4, corresponds to the Hemophilia mutation, indicating the presence of the mutant allele.)
[3]Scanning the AAT-Z mutation.

cles are retrieved making polar body removal (PBR) feasible. Following polar body removal and genetic analysis, one out of four oocytes can be fertilized and transferred. In addition, for the 50% of oocytes with heterozygous polar bodies, the genotype of the oocyte could be determined by aspiration of the second polar body.

In order to apply PBR for preconception genetic diagnosis, the possible detrimental effect of PBR on fertilization and preimplantation development is being studied by careful evaluation of the outcome in each case, including those cases where embryos were predicted to be affected (Verlinsky, 1991).

Polar body removal was performed on over a hundred oocytes retrieved from women who were carriers for cystic fibrosis (CF), alpha-1-antitrypsin deficiency, and hemophilia A. No significant decrease was observed in the fertilization rate for

Table V Preimplantation Genetic Analysis of Alpha-1-Antitrypsin Deficiency

	Normal	Heterozygous	Affected	Failed PCR	Total
Oocyte after PBR	13	27	6	5	51
Blastomere after PBR	9	9	0	1	19
Oocyte Unfertilized	5	7	5	1	18

Table VI Follow-up of the Polar Body Diagnosis in Preimplantation Genetic Diagnosis of Alpha-1-Antitrypsin Deficiency

Oocyte number	PB genotype	Pronucleus	Blastomere genotype	Oocyte Aspiration	Transfer
1	Z/Z[1]	2	—	—	N[3]
2	M/Z	0	—	M/M	N
3	M/Z	0	—	M/Z	N
4	M/Z	0	—	M/M	N
5	M/Z	0	—	M/M	N
6	M/Z	0	—	No amp	N
7	M/Z	2	—	—	Y[4]
8	M/Z	0	—	—	N
9	M/Z	2	—	—	N
10	No amp[2]	2	—	—	N
11	No amp	3	—	—	N
12	M/Z	2	M/Z	—	N
13	M/Z	0	—	—	N
14	No amp	4	—	—	N
15	M/M	2	No amp	—	N
16	Z/Z	2	M/Z	—	N
17	Z/Z	2	M/Z	—	N
18	Z/Z	2	M/Z	—	N
19	M/Z	3	M/Z	—	N
20	M/Z	0	—	Z	N
21	M/Z	0	—	Z	N
22	Z/Z	0	M/M	—	N
23	Z/Z	2	—	—	Y
24	Z/Z	2	M/Z	—	N
25	Z/Z	2	M/Z	—	N
26	M/Z	2	M/M	—	N
27	M/Z	0	—	M	N
28	M/Z	2	M/M	—	N
29	M/M	0	—	Z	N
30	M/Z	2	M/M	—	N
31	Z/Z	0	—	Z	N
32	M/M	0	—	Z	N
33	M/Z	0	—	M/Z	N
34	M/Z	0	—	M/Z	N
35	M/Z	2	M/M	—	N
36	M/M	2	M/Z	—	N
37	M/M	2	M/Z	—	N
38	M/Z	0	—	M/Z	N

(Continued)

Table VI Follow-up of the Polar Body Diagnosis in Preimplantation Genetic Diagnosis of Alpha-1-Antitrypsin Deficiency *(Continued)*

Oocyte number	PB genotype	Pronucleus	Blastomere genotype	Oocyte Aspiration	Transfer
39	Z/Z	2	—	—	Y
40	Z/Z	2	—	—	Y
41	M/M	0	—	M/Z	N
42	No amp	2	M/M	—	N
43	M/Z	0	—	Damaged during PBR	N
44	M/Z	0	—	M/Z	N
45	No amp	0	—	Damaged during PBR	N
46	M/Z	2	M/M	—	N
47	Z/Z	0	—	M/M	N
48	M/Z	0	M/M	—	N
49	M/Z	2	M/M	—	N
50	Z/Z	0	—	Damged during PBR	N
51	Z/Z	0	—	M/Z	N

[1]Z/Z = homozygous abnormal, Z/M = heterozygous, M/M = homozygous normal
[2]No amplification
[3]No
[4]Yes

oocytes following PBR, the percentage of embryos entering cleavage being the same in oocytes subjected to PBR as in control oocytes (Table I). Also, there was no increase in the percentage of polyspermic embryos in the PBR oocytes. The absence of significant deleterious effects of PBR on fertilization and preembryonic development is in agreement with the assumption that the first polar body does not play a role in embryo development.

Possible detrimental effects of PBR in the period after cleavage are also being studied by culturing the affected embryos to the blastocyst stage (Verlinsky et al., 1991a). In these cases, blastomere biopsy (BB) was performed in addition to PBR, either to confirm the diagnosis, in cases where the polar body appeared to be normal, or to select unaffected embryos for transfer, if the polar body appeared to be heterozygous. Table II shows the effect of each procedure separately, as well as the combined effect of PBR and BB. Blastomere biopsy was performed in 62 cases following PBR and lead to the identification of 32 embryos for transfer. From the remaining 30 embryos, 28 developed to the blastocyte stage—a highly acceptable ratio for human embryos—suggesting that there was no detrimental effect of the micromanipulations and biopsy on preimplantation development.

A study of the reliability of preconception genetic diagnosis is of great importance

Table VII Preimplantation Genetic Analysis of Hemophilia A

	Normal	Heterozygous sexed M/F	Affected PCR	Blast	Failed	Total
Oocyte after PBR	21	19	9	—	13	62
Blastomere after PBR	0	2[1]	2[1]	7/15	3	25

[1]Also sexed from the same biopsied blastomere. PCR = Polymerase chain reaction.

before it can be applied in clinical practice. A clinical trial of this approach has been recently carried out, and included the following 12 couples who volunteered to participate: 5 couples at risk for conceiving a child with CF, 1 couple at risk for conceiving a child with alpha-1-antitrypsin deficiency, 1 couple at risk for conceiving a child with hemophilia, and 1 couple at risk for Tay-Sach's disease (Table III).

Table IV presents the results of genetic analysis of 145 polar bodies: 22 for the delta-F508 mutation of CF, 62 for hemophilia (XbaI polymorphism in the factor VIII gene), 51 for alpha-1-antitrypsin deficiency (AAT-ZZ), and 10 for Tay-Sach's disease (TSD). Successful analysis has been achieved in 18 polar bodies for delta-F508 mutation (82%), in 49 for hemophilia (79%), in 46 for -1-antitrypsin deficiency (90%), and in 7 for TSD (70%). This experience is described in more detail in the section on DNA analysis of polar bodies and preembryos.

In brief, successful analyses of polar bodies for delta-F508 mutation, showed that 5 oocytes were normal (28%), 5 were heterozygous (28%), and 8 were abnormal (44%).

Of the successful analyses of polar bodies for hemophilia, 21 (43%) appeared to be normal, i.e., showed the presence of the HbaI polymorphic site corresponding to the normal gene in this family, 9 (18.4%) were lacking XbaI polymorphic site, indicating that the corresponding oocyte was normal, and 19 (39%) were heterozygous, containing both XbaI polymorphic sites.

Of 46 successful analyses of polar bodies for AAT-Z mutation, 6 (13%) were identified as normal AAT-M and 27 (59%) were heterozygous (AAT-ZM), while 13 (28%) appeared to be affected (AAT-Z) indicating that corresponding oocytes are free from the abnormal gene.

Of 7 successful analyses of polar bodies for TSD, 3 were abnormal indicating that the corresponding oocytes are normal, 2 were normal and 2 were heterozygous.

Unfortunately, there is not much information on confirmation of the diagnosis following PBR, as many of the transferred embryos did not implant. However, some of the oocytes subjected to PBR were followed-up by blastomere biopsy or other possible sampling to demonstrate the reliability of diagnosis. The data on the follow

Table VIII Follow-up of the Polar Body Diagnosis in Preimplantation Diagnosis of Hemophilia A

Oocyte	Polar Body	Pronucleus	Blastomere Genotype	Transfer
1	7.3–7.4	2	—	N
2	7.4–7.4	2	—	N
3	7.3–7.3	0	—	N
4	7.3–7.4	2	—	N
5	7.4–7.4	0	—	N
6	7.3–7.4	0	—	N
7	7.3–7.3	3	—	N
8	7.4–7.4	2	—	Y
9	7.4–7.4	1	—	Y
10	No amp	1	—	N
11	7.3–7.3	2	—	N
12	No amp	2	Male	N
13	7.3–7.4	0	—	N
14	No amp	2	—	
15	7.4–7.4	2	—	
16	7.4–7.4	2	—	Y
17	7.4–7.4	2	—	N
18	No amp	2	Male	N
19	No amp	2	Female	N
20	7.3–7.3	2	Female	N
21	7.4–7.4	2	—	Y
22	7.4–7.4	2	—	Y
23	No amp	2	Female	N
24	No amp	2	Female	N
25	7.3–7.4	2	Male	N
26	7.4–7.4	2	No amp	N
27	7.3–7.3	2	Female	N
28	7.4–7.4	2	Female	N
29	7.3–7.4	2	Female	N
30	7.3–7.4	2	Male	N
31	7.3–7.4	2	Female	Y
32	7.3–7.4	2	Female	Y

(Continued)

Table VIII Follow-up of the Polar Body Diagnosis in Preimplantation Diagnosis of Hemophilia A *(Continued)*

Oocyte	Polar Body	Pronucleus	Blastomere Genotype	Transfer
33	7.3–7.4	2	Female	Y
34	7.3–7.4	2	Male	N
35	7.3–7.4	2	Female	Y
36	7.3–7.4	0	—	N
37	7.3–7.4	0	Male	N
38	7.3–7.4	0	—	N
39	7.3–7.4	2	Female	N
40	No amp	2	Female 7.3–7.4	N
41	7.3–7.4	5	—	N
42	No amp	2	No amp	N
43	7.4–7.4	2	—	Y
44	7.4–7.4	0	No amp	N
45	7.4–7.4	0	—	N
46	7.3–7.3	2	Male 7.4	N
47	7.4–7.4	3	—	N
48	7.3–7.4	2	—	N
49	Technical Problem	2	Female	N
	No res.	0	7.3	N
50	7.3–7.3	0	—	N
51	7.4–7.4	0	—	N
52	7.4–7.4	0	—	N
53	7.3–7.3	2	Male 7.4	N
54	No amp	0	—	N
55	7.4–7.4	0	—	N
56	7.4–7.4	2	—	Y
57	7.3–7.3	2	—	N
58	No amp	0	Female	N
59	7.4–7.4	2	—	Y
60	No amp	1	—	N
61	7.4–7.4	2	—	Y
62	7.3–7.3	0	—	N

up of the polar body diagnosis of CF was as follows. Two oocytes predicted to be heterozygous by polar body analysis did not fertilize and were analyzed and found to have the two different alleles, thus confirming the polar body analysis for the delta-F508 mutation. Four oocytes predicted to be homozygous delta-F508 by polar body analysis resulted in preembryos whose genotypes were determined by blastomere biopsy to be heterozygous. In addition, of five oocytes predicted to be heterozygous for delta F-508, four resulted in embryos whose genotypes were determined by blastomere biopsy to be homozygous normal, and one was heterozygous (Verlinsky et al., 1991b).

The follow-up of the preconception diagnosis for alpha-1-antitrypsin deficiency is shown in Tables V and VI. Preconception diagnosis was confirmed by blastomere biopsy in 17 cases where oocytes were predicted to be affected or heterozygous, and by oocyte aspiration in 17 cases where no fertilization was observed.

Reliability of diagnosis in cases of hemophilia was monitored mainly by blastomere biopsy and gender determination using X- and Y-specific primers, except in two cases where XbaI polymorphism in blastomeres confirmed the polar body diagnosis (Tables VII and VIII). Finally, one of the embryos predicted to be unaffected by PBR for hemophilia A spontaneously aborted due to trisomy 16 and appeared to have no mutant allele in the X chromosome, thus confirming the polar body diagnosis.

As can be seen from Tables IX and X, the experience with preconception diagnosis of TSD is much smaller; however, there was an opportunity to confirm polar body diagnosis by genotyping of two unfertilized oocytes and of two embryos, one of which was predicted to be affected. The other, though predicted to be normal by polar body analysis, appeared to be heterozygous due to triploidy after fertilization.

Although in preconception genetic diagnosis the genotype of the oocyte is extrapolated from the opposite diagnosis of the polar body, there have been no misdiagnoses so far. This suggests that there might be no need for further information about embryos whose first polar bodies were found to be homozygous for the

Table IX Preimplantation Genetic Analysis of Tay-Sach's Disease

	Normal	Heterozygous	Affected PCR	Failed	Total
Oocyte after PBR	3	2	2	3	10
Blastomere after PBR	1	2	1	4	8
Oocyte Unfertilized	2	0	0	0	2

PCR = polymerase chain reaction

abnormal recessive gene. For either a recessive or a dominant gene carried by the mother, fertilization of such oocytes will result in an unaffected fetus. Analysis of the second polar body may also make possible the utilization of heterozygous oocytes, leading in fact to identification of all oocytes which contain the unaffected gene. However, in recessive diseases, 50% of oocytes containing the abnormal gene will be fertilized with sperm carrying the normal gene and will be unaffected. Therefore, polar body analysis will not be able to identify all normal embryos, the remaining unaffected embryos have to be identified by embryo biopsy and genotype analysis during preimplantation development, as described below.

Preimplantation Genetic Analysis by Blastomere Biopsy

In spite of some clear advantages of preconception genetic diagnosis, it will not always be possible to establish a genetic diagnosis of the embryo by PBR, due to a number of factors, for example:

1. Paternal alleles cannot be analyzed.
2. The test might not be efficient for telomeric loci since crossing-over will occur with high frequency leading to the heterozygous state of the polar body.
3. Gender determination is not possible.

Table X Follow-up of the Polar Body Diagnosis in Preimplantation Diagnosis of Tay-Sach's Disease

Oocyte number	Polar body genotype	Pronucleus	Blastomere genotype	Oocyte aspiration	Transfer	Additional biopsy
1	I/N	2	No amp		No	I/N
2	No amp	2	N/N		Yes	
3	No amp	2	No amp		No	I/N
4	I/N	2	No amp		No	I/I
5	N/N	2	No results[1]		No	
6	No amp	0	I/N[2]		No[3]	
7	I/I	3	I/N		No	
8	N/N[2]	2	I/I[2]		No	
9	I/I	0	—	N/N	No	
10	I/I	0	—	N/N	No	

[1]Technical problems
[2]I/I = homozygous affected, I/N = heterozygous, N/N = homozygous normal
[3]Delayed cleavage

Table XI Preimplantation Genetic Analysis to Determine Sex (Fragile X, Lesch-Nyhan's Syndrome, Hemophilia A)

	Male	Female	Failed PCR	Add. Biopsy (M/F/Failed PCR)	Total PCR
Blastomere biopsy only	14	20	20[1]	7/7/3	71

[1]Three embryos failed amplification on two biopsies each.

In addition, the fact that in PBR the genotype of the oocyte is inferred rather than directly determined, is an additional weakness. In the above situations blastomere biopsy becomes an important complement to PBR.

Embryo biopsy is performed at the 4- to 8-cell stage, and the microtools used for embryo biopsy are the same as those for PBR, except for minor modifications (described in detail in the section on embryological aspects). As mentioned, PGD by blastomere biopsy was first demonstrated for X-linked disorders, and performed by gender determination of human embryos (Handyside et al. 1989, 1990). Eight couples known to be at risk of transmitting various X-linked diseases participated in this clinical trial, including those at risk for X-linked mental retardation, Lesch-Nyhan's syndrome, adrenoleukodystrophy, retinitis pigmentosa, hereditary sensory motor neurone disease type II, and Duchenne's muscular dystrophy (DMD). Embryo biopsy was performed on day 3, at the 6- to 10-cell stage, and one to three blastomeres from each cleaving embryo were removed. The sequence specific for the Y chromosome was amplified from the biopsied cells for gender determination, while the corresponding biopsied embryos were returned to culture and those diagnosed as females were transferred to achieve a pregnancy. As a result five women became pregnant: three after one treatment cycle, one after two cycles, and one after three cycles. Of 22 biopsied embryos which were transferred, 10 implanted; this suggests a 45% implantation rate per embryo transferred. Of 10 embryos implanted, 7 developed to the fetal heart stage. Of these, chorionic villus sampling (CVS) confirmed the embryo biopsy in six of them. The remianing fetus had been misdiagnosed and this pregnancy with a misdiagnosed singleton male was terminated. The six females have all been born, and one set of twins, born July 15, 1990, have already had their second birthday. One of the second set of twins was stillborn but there were no gross abnormalities.

One of the important observations of this study was the exceptionally high success rate in achieving pregnancies following blastomere biopsy. The rate appeared to be twice as high as that in the best in vitro fertilization (IVF) programs. In fact, the study of the viability of the biopsied preembryos did not reveal any detrimental effect due to the above procedures: over 70% of the manipulated embryos reached blastocyst stage, with no significant reduction in cell number and energy substance (glucose and pyruvate) uptake (Hardy et al., 1989a).

The other reported experience of PGD by preembryo biopsy includes couples at risk for conceiving a child with CF, hemophilia A, Lesch-Nyhan's syndrome, and X-linked mental retardation (Verlinsky et al., 1991b; Verlinsky et al., 1992). In the case of CF, blastomere biopsy was mainly used to confirm polar body diagnosis in embryos which were predicted to be affected, or to identify unaffected embryos for transfer, among those embryos which were predicted by polar body analysis to be heterozygous (described in the previous section). However, in one case of blastomere biopsy, when the CF mutation in one of the parents was unknown, preimplantation diagnosis resulted in the transfer of an affected embryo (described in detail in Section VII). Experience with blastomere biopsy for preimplantation diagnosis of the X-linked diseases previously mentioned is presented in Table XI. A total of 71 embryos (from three couples; a total of 11 cycles) were biopsied at the 8-cell stage. As a result of these biopsies, 27 female embryos were identified for transfer, with only three cases in which there was failure of amplification.

Another experience with preimplantation diagnosis, recently reported by Lesko et al. (1991), includes three patients at risk for conceiving a fetus with CF (delta-F508) and one at risk for Lesch-Nyhan's syndrome. From 10 oocytes, recovered from the latter patient, 9 were fertilized, and of these 7 were biopsied and genotyped using the latest developments in DNA amplification. However, only one of the embryos appeared to be normal and was transferred, and no pregnancy was observed. From three patients at risk for CF the following observations were made: there was no embryo of good quality for transfer in one of the patients, in spite of the availability of preimplantation diagnosis; two of five biopsied embryos in the other patient appeared unaffected, but no pregnancy was achieved following their transfer; and, finally, six of 11 oocytes recovered from the third patient were fertilized and biopsied on day 3, two of which appeared to be unaffected and were transferred. As a result one singleton pregnancy is in progress, with the biopsy results to be confirmed by CVS.

A clinical trial for preimplantation diagnosis based on blastomere biopsy has also been started by Cohen and Grifo (personal communication). Their first case was an IVF patient, a carrier of hemophilia A, who has undergone 12 cycles of artificial insemination due to male factor infertility. Thirteen oocytes were obtained, of which 10 were fertilized and biopsied. Genetic diagnosis was successful for eight embryos. Multiple PCR with X- and Y-chromosome-specific coamplification identified four unaffected (female) embryos, three of which were transferrable. Although no pregnancy was observed in this case, it was possible to confirm the diagnosis in the affected embryos, following successful growth of the three of them to the blastocyst stage.

Finally, Handyside has recently initiated a clinical trial of preimplantation diagnosis by blastomere biopsy with the use of an in situ hybridization technique. In this way six treatment cycles were done, in which the decision about the genotype of the embryo was made only if there was a combination of both of X and Y signals. As a result of that preliminary work, one biochemical pregnancy was achieved; the outcomes of other attempts were not clear at the time this section was written (Handyside, 1992 unpublished).

The application of blastomere biopsy complements preconception genetic analysis, which, as mentioned, is not applicable for gender determination and for autosomal recessive conditions when the carrier status of the mother is not available. In addition, blastomere biopsy is performed in all cases, except when PBR reveals that the polar body is homozygous for the defective allele as the corresponding preembryos are transferred. Those preembryos whose polar bodies were normal or heterozygous, and those whose PCR analysis failed weree biopsied at the 4- to 8-cell stage, so that unaffected embryos could be transferred in the same cycle or frozen for a subsequent transfer.

The two above-mentioned approaches to PGD, using PBR and blastomere biopsy, seem to be complementary rather than competing methods. In future clinical practice they could be used to genotype oocytes and preembryos and to confirm preconception genetic diagnosis for autosomal recessive, dominant, and X-linked disorders.

Preimplantation Genetic Analysis by Blastocyst Biopsy

Blastocyst biopsy as a possibility for PGD was first reported in rabbits by Gardner and Edwards (1968). It seems to be the most realistic among other not-yet-realized but potentially possible approaches for PGD in humans. Extensive studies on the development of blastocyst biopsy in human blastocysts have been undertaken by Dokras et al. (1990). Since in the human blastocyst the number of cells increases to over a hundred, the authors were able to remove as many as 10 to 30 cells from IVF embryos for biopsy at this stage, without replacing any of them. Another advantage of this approach is that trophectoderm cells can be biopsied without affecting the inner cell mass, from which the embryo is derived. As the feasibility of the technique for clinical use will obviously depend on possible detrimental effects of the manipulations, the authors have initiated a study, which is now in progress, on the viability of biopsied blastocysts in vitro, using morphological criteria and the patterns of human chorionic gonadotropin (HCG) secretion. Because there was no information on the development of nonmanipulated embryos in vitro for comparison, 36 nonmanipulated human embryos from day 3 to day 14 were investigated. In this study the authors observed hatching in 38% of the blastocysts, with HCG being first identified on day 8, peaking at day 10, and still being detectable in some blastocysts at day 14. For the individual blastocysts, the pattern of HCG secretion correlated with the assessment of morphology (Dokras et al., 1990). The method of trophectoderm biopsy is described in the section on embryological aspects.

Blastocyst biopsy at present may be intiated only through uterine lavage because the proportion of embryos which reaches this stage in IVF programs is very low (Hardy et al., 1989b). Although the potential advantage of blastocyst biopsy is obvious, there has not been any reported attempt to use this approach for PGD of human genetic diseases. Current research on the development of blastocyst biopsy in experimental animals and in man will make it possible to consider the usefulness of blastocyst biopsy not only as an alternative approach for PGD, but also for confirmation of preconception or blastomere genetic analysis, or as a back up procedure if these approaches fail. The prospects for blastocyst biopsy application will also depend on the pregnancy success rate after transfer of blastocysts, a rate which has been reported to be insufficiently high for clinical practice (Dawson et al., 1988; Bolton et al., 1991).

References

Arnheim N, Li H, Cui X (1990): PCR analysis of DNA sequences in single cells: Single sperm gene mapping and genetic disease diagnosis. Genomics 8:415–419.

Arnheim N, Li H, Cui X, Navidi W (1991): Single sperm PCR analysis—implications for preimplantation genetics disease diagnosis. In Verlinsky Y, Kuliev AM (eds): "Preimplantation Genetics." New York: Plenum Press, pp. 121–130.

Bolton VN, Wren ME, Parsons JH (1991): Pregnancies following in vitro fertilization and transfer of human blastocysts. Fert Steril 55:830–832.

Coutelle C, Williams C, Handyside A, Hardy K, Winston R, Williamson R (1989): Genetic analysis of DNA from single human oocytes—a model for preimplantation diagnosis of cystic fibrosis. Br Med J 299:22–24.

Dawson KF, Rutherford AJ, Winston NJ, Subak-Sharpe R, Winston RML (1988): Human blastocyst transfer, is it a feasible proposition? Human Reprod 145:44–45.

Dokras A, Sargent IK, Ross C, Gardner RL, Barlow DH (1990): Trophectoderm biopsy in human blastocysts. Human Reprod 5:821–825.

Gardner RL, Edwards RG (1968): Control of the sex ratio at full term in the rabbit by transferring sexed blastocysts. Nature 218:346–348.

Gordon JW, Gang I (1990): Use of zona drilling for safe and effective biopsy of murine oocytes and embryos. Biol Reprod 42:869–876.

Handyside AH, Kontogianni EH, Hardy K, Winston RML (1990): Pregnancies from biopsied human preimplantation embryos sexed by Y-specific DNA amplification. Nature 344:768–770.

Handyside AH, Pattinson JK, Penketh RJA, Delhanty JDA, Winston RML, Tuddenham EDG (1989): Biopsy of human preimplantation embryos and sexing by DNA amplification. Lancet 1:347–349.

Hardy K, Hooper MAK, Handyside AH, Ruthorfod AJ, Winston RML, Leese HJ (1989a): Non-invasive measurement of glucose and pyruvate uptake by individual human oocytes and preimplantation embryos. Human Reprod 4:188–191.

Hardy K, Handyside AH, Winston RML (1989b): The human blastocyst: Cell number, death and allocation during late preimplantation development in vitro. Development 107:597–604.

Kuliev A, Modell B, Galjaard H (1985): Perspectives in Fetal Diagnosis of Congenital Disorders. Serono Symposia Review No. 8, Roma, Italy:Ares Serono Symposia.

Leonard M, Kirszenbaum M, Cotinot C, Chesne P, Heyman Y, Stinnaakre MG, Bishop C, Delouis C, Baiman M, Fellous M (1987): Sexing bovine embryos using Y chromosome specific DNA probe. Theriogenology 27:248.

Lesko J, Snabes M, Handyside A, Hughes M (1991): Amplification of the cystic fibrosis F508 mutation from single cells: Applications towards genetic diagnosis of the preimplantation embryo. Am J Hum Genet 49(4): 1210.

Li H, Cui X, Arnheim N (1991): Analysis of DNA sequence variation in single cells. Methods: A Companion to Methods in Enzymology 2(1):49–59.

Li H, Gyllensten UB, Cui X, Saiki RK, Erlich HA, Arnheim N (1988): Amplification and analysis of DNA sequences in single human sperm and diploid cells. Nature 335:414–417.

McLaren A (1985): Prenatal diagnosis before implantation: Opportunities and problems. Prenat Diagn 5:85–90.

Monk M, Muggleton-Harris AL, Rawlings E, Whittingham DG (1988): Preimplantation diagnosis of HPRT-deficient male and carrier female mouse embryos by trophectoderm biopsy. Human Reprod 3:377–381.

Monk M, Handyside AH (1988): Sexing of preimplantation mouse embryos by measurement of X-linked gene dosage in a single blastomere. J Reprod Fertil 82:365–368.

Saiki R, Scharf S, Faloona F, Mullis K, Horn G, Erlich H, Arnheim N (1985): Enzymatic amplification of beta-globin genomic sequences and restriction site analysis for diagnosis of sickle cell anemia. Science 230:1350–1354.

Summers PM, Campbell JM, Miller MW (1988): Normal in vivo development of marmoset monkey embryos after trophectoderm biopsy. Human Reprod 3:389–393.

Verlinsky Y (1991): Biopsy of Gametes. In Verlinsky Y, Kuliev AM (eds): "Preimplantation Genetics." New York: Plenum Press, pp. 39–47.

Verlinsky Y, Ginsberg N, Lifchez A, Valle J, Moise J, Strom CM (1990): Analysis of the first polar body: Preconceptual genetic diagnosis. Human Reprod 5:826–829.

Verlinsky Y, Cieslak J, Evsikov S, et al. (1991a): Effect of subsequent oocyte and blastomere biopsy on preimplantation development. 7th Annual Meeting of the ESHRE and Seventh World Congress on IVF and Assisted Procreation. Hum Reprod 6(Suppl 1):136.

Verlinsky Y, Rechitsky S, Cieslak J, et al. (1991b): Reliability of preconception and preimplantation genetic diagnosis. Proceedings of the Eighth International Congress of Human Genetics, Am J Hum Genet Suppl 49(4):22.

Verlinsky Y, Milayeva S, Evsikov S et al. (1992): Preconception and preimplantation diagnosis for cystic fibrosis. Prenat Diagn 12:103–110.

WHO (1984): Perspectives of fetal diagnosis of congenital diseases. WHO unpublished document HMG/Serono/84.4. Available from the WHO Hereditary Disease Program, WHO, Geneva.

CHAPTER 5

Clinical Aspects of Preimplantation Genetic Diagnosis

Aaron Lifchez and Norman Ginsberg

Successful human in vitro fertilization with embryo transfer (IVF-ET) was reported for the first time in 1978 by Steptoe and Edwards. This therapy was originally designed to treat couples who were infertile by virtue of fallopian tube disease that was not corrected by reconstructive surgery or was judged too extensive to warrant an attempt at reconstructive surgery. Over the last 10 years, this technique has been used to treat couples who are infertile for a variety of other reasons as well, and has been recently applied for preimplantation genetic diagnosis (PGD).

In the early days of IVF-ET it was not clear whether patients should be induced to superovulate through the use of ovulation-inducing drugs, or if oocyte retrieval should follow only a nonmedicated cycle. The early successes of Steptoe and Edwards (1978) were obtained with natural cycles. It soon became clear, however, that stimulated cycles offered several advantages that natural cycles did not. These advantages included:

1. Recovery of multiple mature oocytes.
2. More accurate timing of follicle maturation and, therefore, better timing of oocyte retrieval with subsequent improvement in the quality of oocytes.

Although there is presently renewed interest in natural cycles, most IVF-ET programs use stimulated cycles for the above mentioned reasons. The purpose of this chapter is not to describe in detail the clinical aspects of IVF-ET, but rather to present a brief overview relevant to PGD.

Ovarian Stimulation Regimens

Embryos for preimplantation genetic testing can be obtained through uterine cavity lavage after natural conception, since four days after fertilization the embryo floats freely in the uterus and is accessible by flushing the uterine cavity. A possible application of this approach to PGD is described in detail elsewhere (Brambati and Tului, 1990; Brambati and Formigli, 1991). However, because in uterine lavage only one embryo is obtained per cycle, all ongoing programs on PGD use ovarian stimulation and IVF.

Most ovulation induction protocols now include:

1. A combination of clomiphene citrate (CC), human menopausal gonadotropin (HMG), and human chorionic gonadotropin (HCG), or
2. A combination of gonadotropin-releasing hormones (GNRH) analogs, HMG and HCG.

The combination of CC, HMG, and HCG was first demonstrated to be successful in 1967. The value of CC is that it appears to decrease the amount of HMG required in a given cycle. The initiation of the cycle with CC appears to recruit more follicles than HMG alone. One problem that may occur with the use of CC is a premature surge of luteinizing hormone (LH) that forces the cancellation of the cycle in 25% to 35% of cases. Many IVF-ET programs are therefore changing their ovulation induction protocols to include the use of GnRH agonists along with HMG and HCG. By creating a reversible medical state resembling hypophysectomy, ovarian response to HMG and hCG generally becomes more predictable. With pituitary suppression there cannot, as a rule, be a premature surge of LH and therefore one of the common causes of cycle cancellation is eliminated.

The use of gonadotropin-releasing hormone (GNRH) agonists is particularly valuable when inducing superovulation in women who are 40 years of age or older. The quality of cycles, in terms of quality and quantity of oocytes retrieved is consistently better in this group of women when GnRH agonists are used. The only disadvantage that we, as well as others, have observed when using GnRH agonists, is that more HMG is required and the duration of therapy is often longer. This significantly increases the cost of IVF. Side effects from GnRH agonists are minimal.

During the administration of ovulation-inducing drugs, it is imperative to monitor the patient closely. This insures that the potential for recovering multiple mature oocytes is maximized while the risk to the patient of severe ovarian hyperstimulation is minimized. By monitoring the patient carefully, HCG can be administered at the optimum time, and oocyte retrieval can be scheduled accordingly. Approximately 36 hours after the administration of HCG a mature oocyte has resumed its meiotic process, which results in the extrusion of the first polar body, and a mature oocyte can therefore be retrieved.

During ovulation induction, oocyte quantity and quality is monitored by serial vaginal ultrasound studies and serial determinations of plasma 17-estradiol. With ultrasound one can monitor both follicle number and size. The diameter of a mature follicle varies depending on which ovulation induction protocol was used. The maturity of each follicle should be reflected by a plasma estradiol level of 250–300 pg/ml.

In addition to monitoring oocyte maturation with estradiol levels and ultrasound assessment of follicle size, each cycle is monitored with determinations of LH and progesterone levels. Impending ovulation is detected by an initial rise in progesterone level as well as by the onset of the LH surge that ultimately triggers ovulation. Prior to the use of GNRH agonists, in fully 25% to 30% of cycles were canceled by a premature effort to ovulate, which was characterized by an unexpected rise in LH and progesterone levels.

Oocyte Retrieval

Historically several methods have been used for oocyte retrieval. The oocytes are recovered by aspiration, and the procedure may include:

1. Laparoscopy.
2. Ultrasound guided transabdominal, transvesical, and transvaginal manipulations.
3. Laparotomy.

At present the most frequently employed technique for oocyte retrieval is transvaginal aspiration under ultrasound guidance, which was first described in 1984 by Dellenbach et al. This procedure is generally done under local anesthesia and intravenous sedation, in order to eliminate both the added risk and cost of general anesthesia (Dellenbach et al., 1984; Feichtinger et al., 1986). In addition, it does not require an operating room and, therefore, does not have to compete for time on a busy surgical schedule. With experience an IVF team can accomplish well over 98% of its retrievals using this approach.

The simplest system for follicle aspiration involves the use of a 35-cm 17-gauge needle attached to a 20-cc syringe with a leur lock. More complex systems involve the use of a double-lumen needle with one channel attached to a vacuum pump and the other to an irrigating solution. The needle passes through a needle guide attached to the vaginal ultrasound probe. Software in the ultrasound system displays the path that the needle will follow as the operator advances it. The procedure used in our program is presented below in brief and is the same in both IVF-ET and PGD.

Follicle aspiration is scheduled for 34 hours after the administration of hCG. The patient is asked to arrive for the procedure having eaten no more than a light breakfast. A quick abdominal ultrasound scan is done to make certain that enough follicles are still present. The patient then empties her bladder. Following that an intravenous line (IV) is started, a blood pressure cuff is attached, and the patient is placed in the dorso-lithotomy position. Analgesics are then administered through the IV, the patient is draped, and a sterile field is created. A speculum is inserted into the vagina which is then cleansed with sterile saline, and a topical anesthetic is sprayed on the vaginal vault. Several minutes later the lateral vaginal fornices are infiltrated with a total of 10 cc of 1% Xylocaine.

The vaginal probe is then prepared in a sterile fashion, the needle guide is attached to it and the probe and guide are inserted into the vagina. A follicle is identified and the aspirating needle is guided into it. After puncturing the follicle, its contents are aspirated and delivered to the laboratory which is in an adjacent room. If an oocyte is not recovered, the follicle is then irrigated with 3 cc of media and then reaspirated. The process is repeated until an oocyte is retrieved or a judgement is made that it is unlikely than an oocyte will be retrieved. As long as granulosa cells are identified in the fluid aspirated from a follicle, an attempt will continue to retrieve an oocyte before moving on to the next follicle. This process is repeated until all mature follicles have been aspirated. After all follicles have been aspirated, fluid in the cul-de-sac is aspirated and examined. Occasionally an oocyte that was not recovered in the initial aspiration can be found in the cul-de-sac fluid. Finally, follicular fluid recovered from follicles yielding mature oocytes is returned to the cul-de-sac. The procedure generally take from 30 to 60 minutes. During the procedure a nurse monitors the patient's vital signs and administers additional analgesic as necessary.

Generally our patients are able to return home 1 to 2 hours after the procedure is completed. Prior to discharge, one last ultrasound examination is performed to make certain that there is no evidence of significant bleeding from the ovaries at the sites of follicle aspiration.

Embryo Transfer

The number and quality of oocytes retrieved varies with each patient and indeed may vary in the same patient from cycle to cycle. In traditional IVF, the oocytes are inseminated within 6 hours of aspiration. On the following day fertilization should be evident from the development of zygotes. If development continues properly, on the next day embryos of two to six cells are present. Up to three or four embryos are placed back in the patient's uterus at this time, using a special transfer catheter that is passed transvaginally through the cervix into the uterus. Embryo transfer is without significant patient discomfort and requires no analgesia. The embryo transfer is accomplished, generally, with the patient in the dorsal lithotomy position. Following the transfer, the patient remains in this position for approximately 30 minutes. She is then kept at bed rest in the supine position for an additional 2 hours, after which she is discharged. At the time of discharge the patient is advised to "take it easy" for the remainder of the day. After embryo transfer, IVF programs treat patients with exogenous progesterone and/or HCG. Twelve days after embryo transfer a HCG level is obtained to determine whether or not the patient is pregnant.

The success rate for IVF-ET has slowly risen over the last 10 years. It varies greatly from program to program, with older more established programs generally handling a greater number of cases, and with a greater degree of success. Success rates will, however, vary greatly, depending on the couples undergoing the procedure. Women over the age of forty have a poorer success rate, as do couples with male factor infertility.

Success rate is now most commonly reported as the "take-home baby" rate. This represents the number of live deliveries per 100 successful oocyte retrievals. The Society of Assisted Reproductive Technology (SART) IVF-ET Registry reports this rate to be 14% for the calendar year 1990 (SART, 1992).

As a rule three or four embryos, if available, are transferred with each cycle. Should there be more embryos they are generally frozen; these can then be made available for transfer in a later cycle. The take-home baby rate using frozen-thawed embryos approaches that of cycles in which "fresh" embryos are transferred, and was reported by SART to be 9% for the calendar year 1990. Embryos can be successfully cryopreserved from the second pronuclear stage up to and including the blastocyst stage. It appears that the outcome of pregnancies resulting from the transfer of frozen-thawed embryos is no different than that for pregnancies resulting from the transfer of fresh embryos.

Possible Complications Following IVF-ET and PGD

When looked at from both the obstetrical and gynecological point of view, PGD is associated with the same risks to both the mother and child as those that may result from traditional IVF-ET. Despite the obvious benefits that can be attained through this technology there are potential pitfalls that need to be considered. Complications may occur in connection with:

1. Ovulation induction.
2. Oocyte retrieval.
3. Embryo transfer.
4. Pregnancy, labor, or delivery.

When PGD is combined with IVF-ET there is an even greater need to collect more ova in a cycle, since about 50% of them may be unsuitable for fertilization or transfer.

In an effort to achieve this end GNRH agonists are commonly used to downregulate the pituitary gland. This generally results in the production of more mature ova at one time, and in addition, prevents a premature release of luteinizing hormone. This in turn has the advantage that there are fewer cancelled cycles; however, the cost of the treatment cycle increases since more medication is generally required.

Ovarian hyperstimulation is the only reported complication which is related to the use of ovulation-inducing medications. It can be a serious and even a life-threatening condition, although its incidence is less than 0.5%. It develops only following the administration of HCG. In severe cases, patients may develop ascites, pleural effusion, electrolyte derangement, and hypovolemia with associated hypotension, hemoconcentration, and oliguria. Balasch et al., (1990) reported an acute case of prerenal failure and liver dysfunction in a patient undergoing IVF.

Patients that develop a hyperstimulation syndrome may need to be admitted to the hospital for bed rest, with daily weighing, strict monitoring of their bodily intake and output, and frequent attention to their vital signs (Shapiro et al., 1977). There is a need to focus on measurements of the hematocrit, blood urea nitrogen (BUN), creatinine, electrolytes, total protein with albumin–globulin ratio, coagulation studies, and urinary sodium and potassium. Restriction of fluids and salt may be required. Diuretics should be avoided since they can lead to even greater hypovolemia and increased hemoconcentration. Potassium exchange resins may be required when dangerous levels of hyperkalemia develop (Engle et al., 1972).

In the early days of IVF-ET, oocyte retrieval required general anesthesia and operative laparoscopy. Complications then included the possibility of all of those related to the administration of a general anesthetic, and to the procedure of laparoscopy itself. In addition there were the risks related to follicle puncture and resultant ovarian bleeding. With the introduction of transvaginal ultrasound-guided follicle aspiration, the risks related to anesthesia and laparoscopy have been eliminated. Infrequently, ultrasound-guided aspirations can cause ovarian bleeding that, on very rare occasions, requires surgical intervention. In theory transvaginal aspiration carries with it the added risk of pelvic infection, although in practice we have not seen this complication.

Complications related to embryo transfer are exceptionally infrequent. They include uterine infection and trauma to the wall of the uterus from the embryo transfer catheter.

Finally, once pregnant, the patient is exposed to all potential pregnancy-related complications. Some of these do occur with greater frequency in IVF-ET pregnancies. The risk of spontaneous abortion is greater. Most abortions occurring in IVF-ET pregnancies occur early and do not, as a rule, require surgical intervention. Ectopic pregnancy is another complication that occurs with IVF-ET. The incidence of this complication in IVF-ET pregnancies was reported as 5% (SART, 1992. This rate seems to be highest in women with a previous history of an ectopic pregnancy. This rate is greatly increased over that seen in the general population. In the general population one can expect to see 8.3 ectopic pregnancies per 1,000 (Kitchin et al., 1979).

When IVF is performed, the presence of an intrauterine pregnancy does not exclude the possibility of an associated ectopic pregnancy. This is an important consideration since the death rate from an ectopic pregnancy is 0.8/1,000 (Doyle et al., 1991).

When IVF is used, there are several possible reasons why ectopic pregnancies are seen at a much higher rate than in natural conception. Tubal disease is the most common factor that has been correlated with the development of an ectopic pregnancy. This is similarly the most common indication for IVF. When PGD is the primary indication for IVF-ET, tubal disease is less likely to be present and the incidence of ectopic pregnancy should decrease. As PGD becomes more widely used it will be important to monitor for the incidence of this particular complication.

Supraphysiologic levels of estradiol and progesterone are known to impair normal tubal ciliar motion and proper smooth muscle contractility. This may play a role in the higher incidence of ectopic pregnancies seen in patients that are induced with either Pergonal® or Clomid® (Doyle et al., 1991). These same supraphysiologic levels of estradiol and progesterone will be present when IVF is used for PGD.

The embryo itself may play a role in the development of an ectopic pregnancy. It is known that over half of embryos fail to develop in ectopic pregnancies, although Elias and associates (1981) did not find a higher incidence of chromosomal abnormalities in such pregnancies.

Finally, the volume of fluid that is necessary to complete the embryo transfer may be an additional factor inducing ectopic pregnancy (Martinez et al., 1986), but this should be unchanged with PGD.

Management of an ectopic pregnancy after IVF or PGD may be more complicated since heterotopic pregnancies are more common in this group of patients. Serial monitoring of chorionic gonadotrophins (HCG) will be of no value in an ectopic pregnancy treated laparoscopically in the presence of a heterotopic pregnancy. The use of methotrexate to manage a persistent ectopic in the presence of a heterotopic pregnancy is contraindicated. The surgical treatment of an ectopic pregnancy also puts the remaining fetus at risk of spontaneous abortion from the effects of manipulation or general anesthesia.

Multiple gestations are clearly one of the greatest obstetrical problems associated with IVF and PGD. According to SART (1992), from 3110 babies born overall, 22% of the clinical pregnancies resulted in multiple delivery: 577 twins, 90 triplets 5 quadruplets, and 1 quintuplet.

Most obstetricians have very little experience with the management of pregnancies involving more than two fetuses. To further complicate this situation there are very few data that describe the outcome for large numbers of triplets or quadruplets.

When triplets are studied the average gestational age at delivery is 33.4 to 35 weeks. An interesting observation, made by Ron-El et al. (1981), was that the average length of pregnancy was two weeks longer in multiparous patients. Petrikovsky (1989) reviewed eleven articles on triplets that covered the period from 1978 to 1985 and comprised 714 fetuses. In this large review several factors became apparent. Predicting the neonatal outcome for triplets includes several factors. After gestational age is considered, birth order (in those pregnancies delivered vaginally), fetal sex, and presentation were all important in predicting the neonatal outcome. It appears that the first-born triplet as a rule fares better than its siblings.

Strict guidelines for pregnancy management or mode of delivery of triplets cannot be determined from this review; however, fetal and maternal outcome does seem to depend on the level of prenatal care received. Several measures were associated with the most favorable outcome. These include: hospitalization with bed rest during the second trimester of pregnancy, serial ultrasound examinations for fetal growth, tocolysis, and administration of corticosteroids for the acceleration of fetal lung maturity. Loucopoulos (1982) was able to demonstrate that bed rest increased the time to delivery from 34.3 ±2.9 weeks in the control group (no bed rest) to 35.75 ±3 weeks in the study group.

The complications most commonly seen with triplets are: prematurity with or without ruptured membranes, pregnancy induced hypertension, anemia, and antepartum and postpartum hemorrhage. The perinatal death rate was 21.3% (Petrikovsky et al., 1989).

Obstetrical experience with quadruplets is much less extensive than with triplets, since they are so much rarer. The frequency of quadruplets is one-tenth that of triplets and, therefore, there is even less data available for study. With the use of detailed medical questionnaires, Collins (1990) surveyed 71 quadruplet pregnancies through The Triplet Connection, a support group for mothers with supermultiples. Over half of the study group was comprised of pregnancies that occurred either in 1988 or the first 6 months of 1989. This study is particularly important since it reflects the effects of current neonatal management.

Early bed rest began at 16.7 weeks and was either complete or partial at that time. The average time of bed rest was 13.1 weeks, with a range of 4 to 24 weeks. Dietary intake was a problem during the first trimester of pregnancy because of hyperemesis, and later, after 26 weeks because of extreme abdominal distention. Despite this, the average weight gain was 45.8 pounds.

Cervical cerclage was utilized in 10 patients because of early cervical effacement. These patients delivered at a mean gestational age of 31.2 weeks, which was not significantly different from those that did not undergo a cerclage. This was contradictory to the findings of Goldman et al. (1989), who utilized it with triplets and quadruplets. Goldman found that the mean age at delivery in patients that had a cerclage was 35 weeks, as opposed to those without that delivered at 30.7 weeks of gestation ($p<0.01$).

Premature labor complicated 70 of 71 pregnancies. In the one patient without premature labor, three stillborn infants and one live one were delivered at 38 weeks.

Tocolysis was used in 83% of pregnancies with a mean onset of premature labor at 24.5 weeks. Although premature labor began at 24.5 weeks of gestation, delivery occurred an average of 7 weeks later, at 31.4 ± 3.6 weeks. Sixty-seven percent of the deliveries occurred after 31.4 weeks, with clustering between 31 and 35 weeks. Eighty-seven percent delivered after 28 weeks.

Thirty-three neonatal deaths occurred in 268 live births (12.3%). Twenty-four of the infants were born before 28 weeks, and 8 were delivered between 28 and 30 weeks of gestation. These results show that if the pregnancy can be carried to 28 weeks of gestation there is a 93% chance of survival; over 85% of these pregnancies reached this mark. The risk of stillbirth begins at 32 weeks when linear growth falls off. After 34 weeks of gestation the fetuses become significantly growth retarded, intrauterine deaths increase, and no neonatal deaths occurred. Delivery at 34 weeks should be considered if the risks involved warrant it.

Multifetal pregnancy reduction and selective fetal termination is a first trimester procedure usually carried out in a pregnancy with three or more fetuses, and designed to increase the chances of survival of the remaining fetuses. To many, the ethical issues involved are somewhat different from those involved in abortion. As PGD is a technique designed primarily to avoid these kinds of considerations, special diligence should be exercised to prevent large multigestations. However, some multifetal gestations will inevitably occur despite the best of intentions, skill, and equipment. For example, Buvat (1990) reported that 2.3% of patients undergoing IVF and gamete intrafallopian transfer (GIFT) in France had a multifetal reduction in 1989.

Early Experience in Preimplantation Genetics

Initial expectations regarding the successful application of IVF-ET technologies to preimplantation genetics were that with PGD it would be easier to obtain large numbers of mature oocytes and to achieve better take-home baby rates following embryo transfer than with IVF-ET alone. These expectations were based on the fact that patients undergoing IVF-ET for purposes of preimplantation genetics were, as a group, younger than typical IVF-ET patients, and had no history of infertility which, of course, is the common denominator of all other IVF-ET patients. However, our experience shows the preimplantation genetics patients have the same "take-home baby" rate as do IVF-ET patients in general. This rate does not vary with the type of preimplantation genetic testing, whether it be by polar body or blastomere biopsy.

PGD is still in the investigational phase of development (Verlinsky et al., 1990). All patients need to be counselled that confirmation of results during pregnancy is essential to detect any error that might have occurred in the initial analysis. This analysis should be done sufficiently early in gestation that the patient may be able to undergo an abortion or treatment depending upon the circumstances. As PGD cases may be associated with multigestations, confirmation of the analysis is more complicated (Handyside et al., 1990), since it is essential that each individual fetus is separately diagnosed. In such cases the placentas may become fused, making it complicated to differentiate the portions of the placentas belonging to each fetus. Care must be taken to describe in great detail the location of each fetus that is sampled so that there is no confusion later if one needs to consider a selective reduction. On the rare occasions that it may not be possible to determine which portion of placenta belongs to which fetus, amniocentesis should be utilized. Preliminary data suggests that, in twins, there is no increased risk associated with CVS compared to amniocentesis, but for gestations with larger numbers of fetuses there is not enough data to derive a conclusion.

Whether PGD will lead to an increased incidence of congenital malformations is still an unanswered question. According to the data reported at the 7th World Congress on In Vitro Fertilization and Assisted Procreation (Paris, 1991), the incidence of congenital malformations is similar to that of the general population. (Beischer and Mackay, 1986). These results indicated that IVF by itself does not increase the risk for congenital malformation, except for a possible increase in the risk of trisomy 21. More data will be needed in this respect, and this shows the importance of applying cytogenetic methods to exclude the transfer of chromosomally abnormal embryos in IVF and PGD.

References

Balasch J, Carmona K, Llach J, Arroyo V, Jove I, Vanrell JA (1990): Acute prerenal failure and liver dysfunction in a patient with severe ovarian hyperstimulation syndrome. Hum Reprod 5:348–351.

Beischer NA, Mackay EV (eds) (1986): "Obstetrics and the Newborns." London: Bailliere Tindall.

Brambati B, Tului L (1990): Preimplantation genetic diagnosis: A new simple uterine washing system. Hum Reprod 5:448–450.

Brambati B, Formigli L (1991): Uterine lavage for preimplantation genetic diagnosis. In Verlinsky Y, Kuliev AM (eds): "Preimplantation Genetics." New York: Plenum Press, pp. 165–174.

Buvat J, Buvat-Herbaut F, Dancoine F (1990): Bilan des procréations médicalement assistées en France en 1989. Fertilité - contraception - sexualité 18:583–586.

Collins M, Bleyl B (1990): Seventy-one quadruplets: Management and outcome. Am J Obstet Gynecol 162:1384–1393.

Dellenbach P, Nisand I, Moreau L, Feger B, Pulmere C, Gerlinger P, Brun B, Rumpler Y (1984): Transvaginal sonographically controlled ovarian follicle puncture for egg retrieval. Lancet 1:1467.

Doyle M, DeCherney A, Diamond M (1991): Epidemiology and etiology of ectopic pregnancy. Obstet Gynecol Clin North Am. 18:1–17.

Elias S, LeBeau M, Simpson JL, Maryian AO (1981): Chromosomal analysis of ectopic human conceptuses. Am J Obstet Gynecol 141:698–703.

Engle T, Jewelewicz R, Dyrenfurth I, Speroff L, Vande Wiele RL (1972): Ovarian hyperstimulation syndrome: Report of a case with notes on pathogenesis and treatment. Am J Obstet Gynecol 112:1052–1060.

Feichtinger W, Kemeter P (1986): Transvaginal sector scan sonography for needle guided transvaginal follicle aspiration and other applications in gynecologic routine and research. Fertil Steril 45:722–725.

Goldman G, Dicker D, Peleg D, Goldman J (1989): Is elective cerclage justified in the management of triplets and quadruplet pregnancy? Aust NZ J Obstet Gynaecol 29:9–12.

Handyside A, Kontogianni E, Hardy K, Winston R (1990): Pregnancy from biopsied human preimplantation embryos sexed by Y specific DNA amplification. Nature 344:768–770.

Kitchin JD, Wein RM, Nunley WC et al. (1979): Ectopic pregnancy: Current clinical trends. Am J Obstet Gynecol 134:870–876.

Loucopoulos A, Jewelewicz R, Vande Weile R (1982): Multiple gestations in management and delivery. Acta Genet Med Gemellol 31:263–266.

Martinez F, Trounson A (1986): An analysis of factors associated with ectopic pregnancy in human in vitro fertilization program. 45:79–87.

Medical Research International, The Society for Assisted Reproduction Technology (SART) (1989): In vitro fertilization-embryo transfer in the United States. 1987 results from the IVF-ET Registry. Fertil Steril 53:13–19.

Medical Research International, The Society for Assisted Reproduction Technology (SART) (1992): In vitro fertilization-embryo transfer in the United States. 1990 results from the IVF-ET Registry. Fertil Steril 57:15–24.

Petrikovsky B, Vintzileos A (1989): Management and outcome of multiple pregnancy of high fetal order: Literature review. Obstet Gynecol Surv 44:578–584.

Ron-El R, Caspi E, Schreyer P (1981): Triplet and quadruplet pregnancies and management. Obstet Gynecol 57:458.

Shapiro A, Thomas T, Epstein M (1977): Management of hyperstimulation syndrome. 28:237–239.

Steptoe PC, Edwards RG (1978): Birth after preimplantation of a human embryo. Lancet ii:366

Trounson AO, Mohr L (1983): Human pregnancy following cryopreservation, thawing and transfer of an eight-cell embryo. Nature 305:707.

Verlinsky Y, Ginsberg N, Lifchez A, Valle J, Moise J, Strom C (1990): Analysis of the first polar body: Preconceptual genetic diagnosis. Hum Reprod 5:826–829.

CHAPTER 6

Embryological and Technical Aspects of Preimplantation Genetic Diagnosis

Yury Verlinsky and Jeanine Cieslak

It is not the aim of this chapter to describe the basic laboratory techniques used in in vitro fertilization (IVF); nonetheless, one cannot perform preimplantation genetic diagnosis (PGD) without the knowledge and application of these techniques. Therefore, to describe the methodological aspects of PGD, the sequence of events regarding IVF and PGD will be reviewed in brief.

Selection Of Oocytes

Once follicular stimulation has been achieved, human chorionic gonadotropin (HCG) is administered to facilitate oocyte maturation in vivo (extrusion of the first polar body). Approximately 34 hours from the time of HCG administration, oocyte recovery is accomplished by ultrasound guided transvaginal aspiration as described in Chapter 5, this volume.

Upon puncture and aspiration of the mature graafian follicle, the follicular fluid is examined in a 60 × 15 mm petri dish for the presence of an oocyte, using a dissecting microscope. At this time the oocyte is graded according to its cumulus size and density as described in Chapter 8, this volume. We are currently using a 1–2 scale. A grading of 2–2 given to an oocyte would correspond to a large cumulus mass with low cell density, indicative of a mature oocyte (Fig. 1); while a grading of 1–1 would correspond to a small cumulus mass with high cell density, indicative of an immature oocyte (Fig. 2). The expansion of the corona radiata, the appearance of the oocyte,

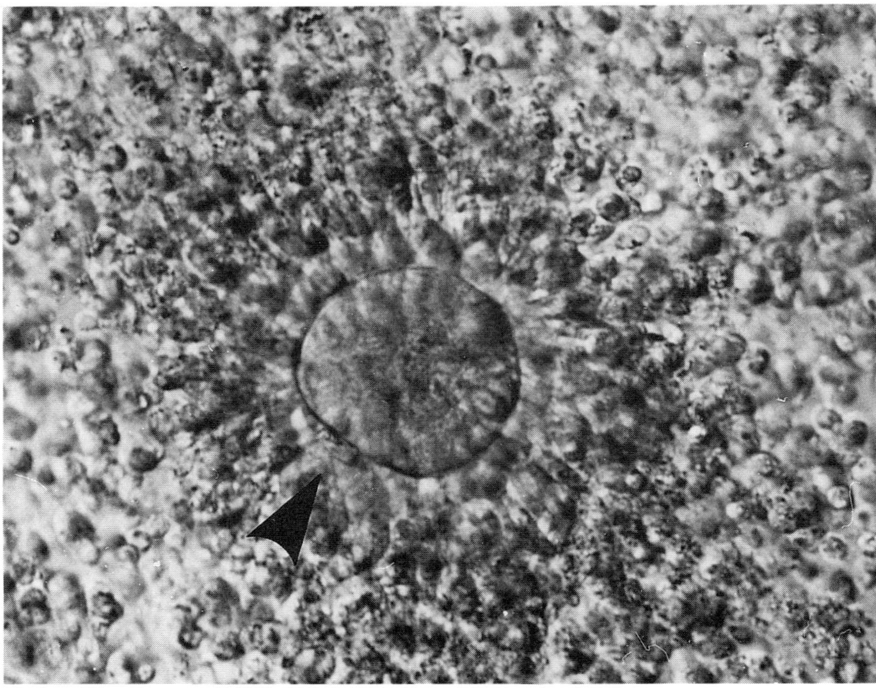

Figure 1 Mature oocyte with expanded corona radiata, first polar body visible (arrowhead) (magnification 400×).

and the presence of the first polar body are also noted. Once graded, the oocyte is washed from its follicular fluid and placed in culture using a 4-well culture dish (Nunc) containing IVF medium (see below). Although there is sometimes asynchrony between cumulus size and density, and the maturity of the oocyte, this grading system gives a good idea of what kind of oocytes we will be working with.

Approximately 2 hours after retrieval, oocytes are removed from culture one at a time and placed in IVF medium containing hyaluronidase (290 U/ml) to liberate them from their cumulus mass. Usually within 1 to 2 minutes the cumulus cells will begin to disperse and can be mechanically removed using an attenuated pipette (Fig. 3A and 3B). Special attention should be paid to thoroughly cleaning the oocytes in order to eliminate the possibility of aspirating corona cells into the micropipette during polar body removal (PBR), which would contaminate the sample with maternal DNA. The hyaluronidase is removed by washing the oocytes in IVF medium; they are then returned to their original culture dishes. At this time, oocyte maturity is determined by the presence of the first polar body (PB), and the oocytes are returned to the

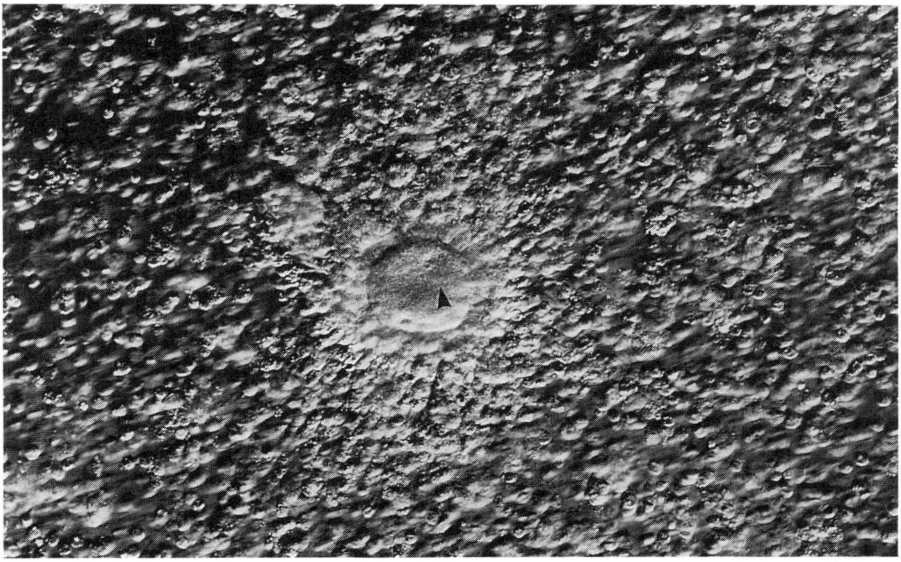

Figure 2 Immature cumulus–oocyte complex, germinal vesicle visible (arrowhead) (magnification 200×).

incubator until micromanipulation is performed. If the oocyte has not extruded its first PB, it is placed back into the incubator to remain undisturbed for a few hours until a second look is taken. Maturation of germinal vesicle oocytes can occur in vitro and generally takes an additional 24 hours until the first PB is extruded. However, the chance of fertilization and development of these oocytes is reduced.

Tool Making and Micromanipulation Setup

There are three main instruments required for tool making: a pipette puller, microforge, and beveler (Fig. 4). The first step in microtool construction is the preparation of microneedles from glass coagulation tubes. This can be done with the use of the Flaming-Brown mechanical pipette puller (Model P-87, Sutter Instrument Co.). The program and heating filament should be adjusted to give the desired length to the tapered end of the microneedle.

The holding pipette (which can also be pulled by hand over a flame in order to receive a longer attenuated tip) is prepared using the DeFronbrune type microforge (Model MF-1, TPI Instruments). Under the control of the microforge stereomicroscope, equipped with eyepiece reticule, the tip of the needle is broken by placing the section of the needle, which approximates 200 µm in diameter, on top of the glass ball which surrounds the heating filament (Fig. 5A). The temperature of the filament is increased until the needle is fused to the glass ball. The power is switched off causing an abrupt decrease in temperature and shrinkage of the heating filament, which, in turn, leads to breakage of the tip of the needle fused to the glass ball (Fig. 5B). Then, the pipette tip is flame-polished by being placed approximately 0.5 mm away from the glass ball while the temperature of the filament is increased to achieve melting of the glass (Fig. 5C). Finally, the attenuated portion of the micropipette is bent by being placed above the glass ball. The filament is heated until the glass begins to soften so that the pipette tip bends by its own weight (approximately a 135° angle) (Fig. 5D). This is done to all microtools, so that they are parallel to one another and to the microscope stage during micromanipulation.

To prepare a partial zona dissection needle (PZD) (Malter and Cohen, 1989) a needle is simply bent on the microforge as for all other microtools. This PZD needle is not connected to the microsyringe system, for there is no opening at the tip.

To prepare beveled micropipettes, the KT Brown type micropipette beveler (Model BV-10, Sutter Instrument Co.) is used. Before the microneedle is attached to the beveler, the plane of beveling is indicated by marking the shoulder of the microneedle with a small dot. This dot should be facing up when the microneedle is

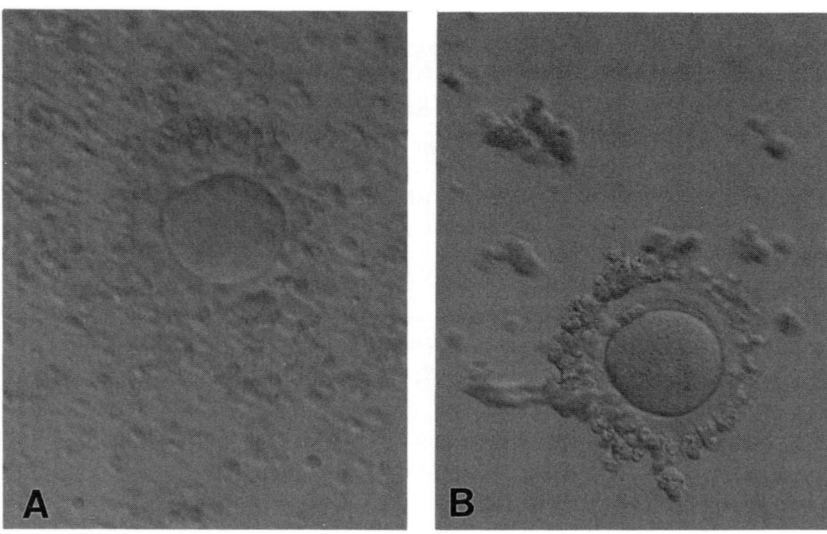

Figure 3 Cleaning of an oocyte from its cumulus cells using hyaluronidase. **A.** After one minute in hyaluronidase cumulus cells begin to disperse (magnification 200×). **B.** Oocyte with remaining corona cells which must be removed mechanically (magnification 200×).

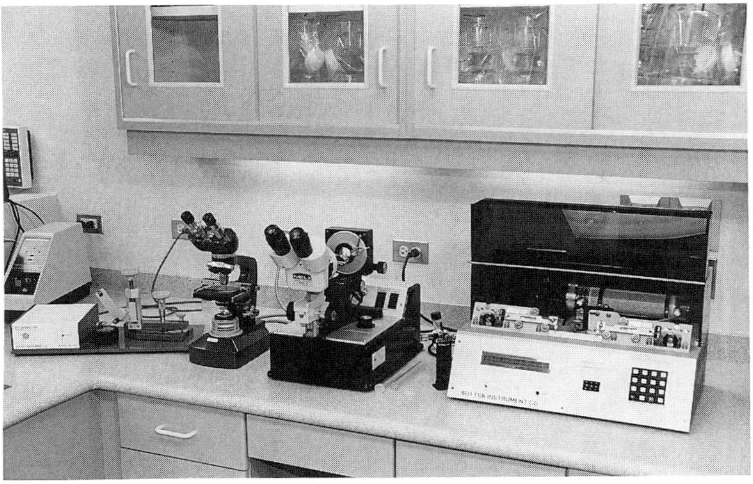

Figure 4 Tool making instruments (from right to left): mechanical pipette puller, microforge, microscope to check diameter of the micropipette, and beveler.

attached to the beveler. The time required for beveling depends upon the pressure applied to the needle, the diameter desired, and the type of glass. This should be determined empirically. Immediately after beveling, the diameter and the quality of beveling are checked under the microscope fitted with an eyepiece reticule, and the needle is thoroughly rinsed with deionized water. The micropipette is bent on the microforge; the dot indicating the plane of beveling should face the operator. For pronucleus removal, the beveled micropipette is siliconized (with Sigmacote, Sigma) to prevent the oocyte plasma membrane from adhering to the glass.

The microtools are stored in a Petri dish (150 × 15 mm). Clay or foam rubber can be used to hold the pipettes in place.

Certain basic equipment is needed for IVF and micromanipulation (see Table I). An incubator is necessary for culturing gametes and embryos at 37°C under 5% CO_2 and 95% O_2, or, as we are currently using, a tri-gas incubator (Heraeus model B5061) which allows for 5% CO_2, 5% O_2, and 90% N_2. A laminar flow hood, such as the Holten LFM 24725, allows for sterility when handling gametes and embryos. This particular model has an immersion heater circulator which makes it possible to control the temperature of the working surface. It also has a dissecting microscope directly built in, to aid in recovery and transfer of oocytes. An inverted microscope (such as the Nikon Diaphot with a stage warmer) for fertilization assessment and micromanipulation is also placed in the hood (Fig. 6). Finally, special measures should be taken to maintain the pH of the culture medium by the use of gas flow meters which control the passage of tri-gas mixture to the working surface of the hood.

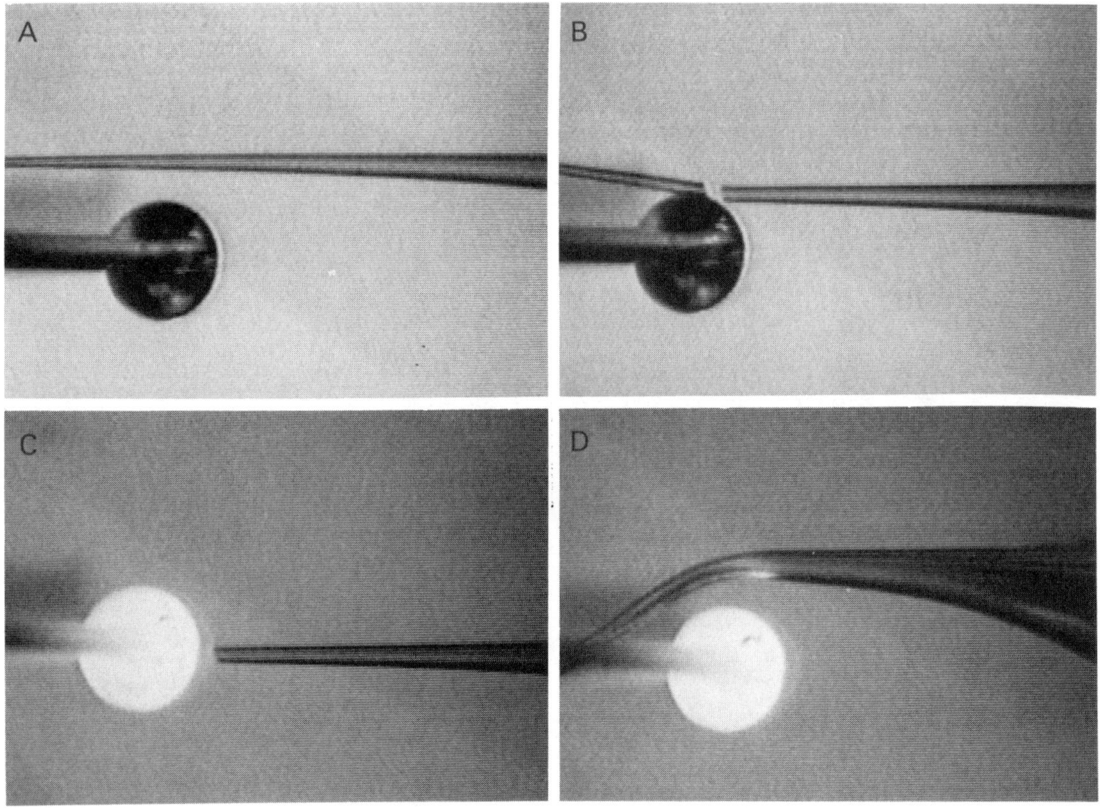
A
B
C
D

Table I Materials Required for In Vitro Fertilization and Micromanipulation

Materials	Source
150 mm coagulation tubes	Fisher #02-667
35×10 mm Petri dishes (Falcon)	Fisher #08-757-100A
60x15 mm Petri dishes (Falcon)	Fisher #08-757-100B
150×15 mm Petri dishes (Falcon)	Fisher #8-757-14
4-well culture dishes (Nunc)	Scientific Supply #176740
50-ml culture flasks (Nunc)	Scientific Supply #NUN163371
200-ml culture flasks (Falcon)	Fisher #10-126-5
Receiver flasks (1 liter) (Nalgene)	Fisher #09-740-25F
0.2 micron filters (1 liter flask) (Nalgene)	Fisher #09-740-26A
0.2 micron acrodisc syringe filters	Fisher #09-730-218
20-cc Becton Dickinson syringe	Fisher #14-823-2B
Sterile Pasteur pipets (5 ¾ in)	In Vitro Scientific Products #601050
1-ml serological pipets (Falcon)	Scientific Supply #BDF7521
5-ml serological pipets (Falcon)	Scientific Supply #BDF7543
10-ml serological pipets (Falcon)	Scientific Supply #BDF7551
25-ml serological pipets (Falcon)	Scientific Supply #BDF7525

For manipulation of gametes and embryos, micromanipulators are mounted on the inverted microscope. The MO202 micromanipulator (Narishige) provides good control of both the beveled and holding micropipettes, as well as convenience and comfort for the operator. However, the less expensive Narishige MN151 can also be used to control the holding pipette. Hydraulic control for the holding pipette can be obtained using the Narishige IM-6 microsyringe and the microsyringe (Stoelting #51218) can be used for the beveled microneedle with slight modification. The micrometer for the Stoelting microsyringe must be connected to the plunger of the microsyringe with epoxy in order for it to aspirate during biopsy. Microsyringes are connected to micropipettes using polyethylene or Teflon tubing (0.040 mm i.d. × 0.070 mm o.d.). The whole hydraulic system including the holding pipette is filled with light paraffin oil; special attention should be paid to eliminate any air bubbles.

Figure 5 Construction of the holding pipette (magnification 400×). **A.** The section of the microneedle which approximates 200 mcm in diameter placed over the glass ball which surrounds the heating filament. **B.** Breakage of the tip of the microneedle fused to the glass ball. **C.** Flame polishing of the micropipette by placing it in front of the glass ball and increasing the temperature of the filament. **D.** Bending of the micropipette by placing it above the glass ball and heating until it bends by its own weight.

Microtools which are needed for biopsy or injection are filled with silicone oil. The viscosity of the silicone oil used will depend on the type of micromanipulation to be performed (Fig. 7).

IVF and PGD Media Preparation

A modified Ham's F-10 medium (see below) is routinely used in our lab for culture and micromanipulation of gametes and embryos. It is a rich medium and, once supplemented, is certainly capable of supporting development to the "hatched" blastocyst stage. A new batch of medium is prepared every 2 weeks and a small aliquot is tested for toxicity with a mouse IVF assay. If over 80% of the oocytes recovered from the mice are fertilized and develop to the blastocyst stage one can assume there are no toxic substances present.

To prepare 1 liter of Ham's F-10 medium, an antibiotic solution is prepared by adding 0.075 g of penicillin G and 0.075 g of streptomycin sulfate to a sterile 1000-ml Nalgene receiver flask. Approximately 900 ml of HPLC (high-pressure liquid chromatography) grade water is added and the antibiotics are dissolved by mixing. To the antibiotic solution, 1 millimole of calcium lactate is added and the solution is

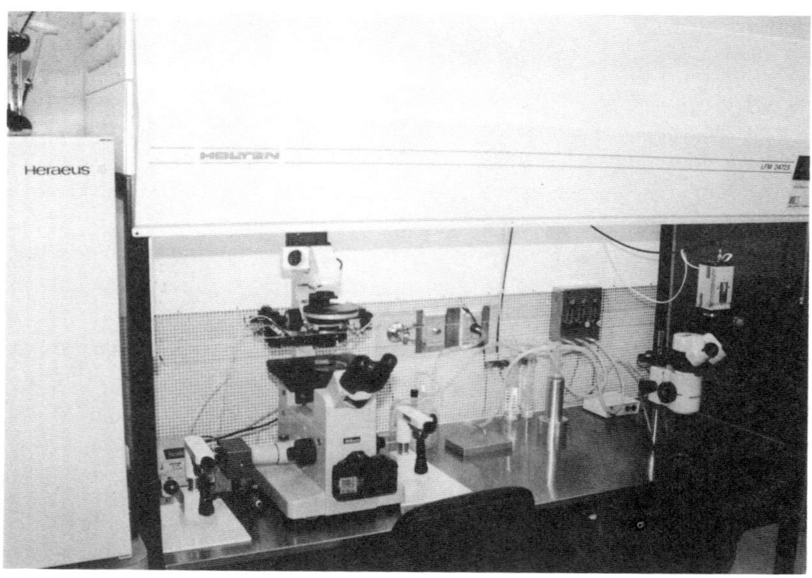

Figure 6 Equipment setup for IVF and PGD.

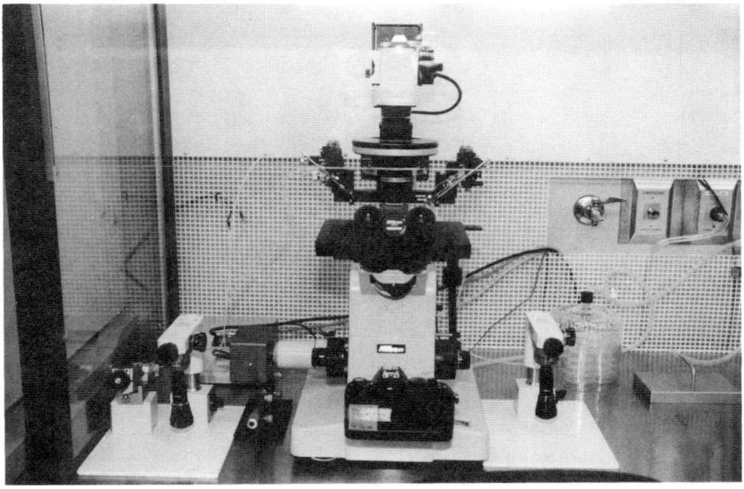

Figure 7 Inverted microscope with mounted micromanipulators.

mixed periodically until complete dissolution of the calcium lactate. This may take 10 to 15 minutes. A packet of Ham's F-10 powder is opened and the contents are emptied into the flask and mixed. The solution will appear orange in color. Finally, 2.1 g of sodium bicarbonate is added and mixed, changing the color of the medium to pink. Upon complete dissolution of the last ingredient, the volume is brought to the 1000ml mark with HPLC grade water and remixed. The osmolarity is checked using an osmometer (Precision Systems) and must be adjusted to 280 ± 2 mOsm. The initial reading is usually between 300 and 315 mOsm. The adjustment can be made using a simple calculation:

$$V = \frac{\text{unadjusted osmolarity - 280 mOsm}}{\text{unadjusted osmolarity}} \times 1000$$

This yields the approximate volume (V) of medium to be exchanged with HPLC grade water. An amount slightly less than the calculated amount should be exchanged, for it is much easier to add an additional few milliliters of HPLC grade water to obtain the desired osmolarity than to try to correct an overdiluted medium.

Once the osmolarity is corrected, the medium is sterile filtered, using a Nalgene 1000 ml 0.2 micron filter unit, and stored at 5°C until needed. A batch of medium can be used for up to 2 weeks.

There are two supplements routinely used in our lab for the final preparation of IVF medium: maternal serum (10%) or synthetic serum replacement (SSR2), and human

Table II Reagents Required for IVF and Micromanipulation

Materials	Source
Paraffin oil	Fisher #0121-4
Silicone oil (12,500 centistokes)	Sigma #DMPS-12M
Silicone oil (60,000 centistokes)	Sigma #DMPS-60M
Sucrose	Sigma #S-9378
Cytochalasin B	Sigma #C-6762
Hyaluronidase	Sigma #H-3506
Sigmacote	Sigma #SL-2
Sodium penicillin-G	Sigma #P-3032
Streptomycin sulfate	Sigma #S-9137
Sodium bicarbonate	Sigma #S-5761
Calcium lactate	Boerhing Biochemical #4272
Ham's F-10 powder	Gibco #430-1200EB
Phosphase buffered saline powder	Gibco #450-1300EC
Heparin 100,000 units	Gibco #820-5077MF
Chromar HPLC water (Mallinckrodt)	Scientific Products #6795-1NY
Human serum albumin	Medi-Cult a/s #001693 (Copenhagen, Denmark)
Synthetic serum replacement 2	Medi-Cult a/s #1004 (Copenhagen, Denmark)

serum albumin (HSA). 40 microliters of both solution A and solution B of the SSR2 and 2 ml of HSA are added to 38 ml of Ham's F-10 medium. Once again the supplemented medium is sterile filtered using a 0.2 micron acrodisc syringe filter.

For PGD, micromanipulation dishes are prepared using Ham's F-10 medium supplemented with SSR2 and HSA. This medium has been found to be consistently free of human DNA.

To prepare paraffin oil both for culturing and for micromanipulations, equal volumes of paraffin oil previously filtered through a Nalgene 1000 ml 0.2 micron filter, and Ham's F-10 medium (unsupplemented) are pipetted into a sterile 200-ml culture flask and capped tightly. The solutions are mixed vigorously by shaking and the cap of the flask is loosened for placement in the incubator for equilibration. After 2 days of incubation, the flask is capped tightly, the solutions are remixed, and the flask is placed back into the incubator for another 3 to 4 days until it can be used. This process of washing the paraffin oil helps reduce the chance of toxic contamination. Phosphate buffered saline (PBS) is prepared for use during recovery of oocytes. If an oocyte is not recovered upon initial aspiration of the follicle, it is necessary to flush

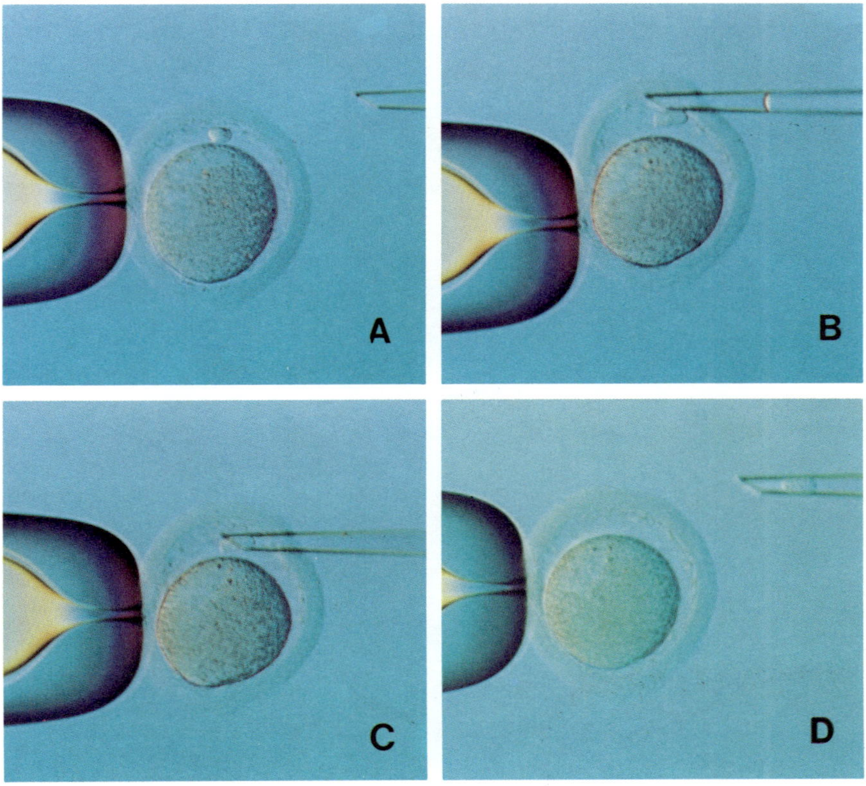

Figure 8 Polar body removal (magnification 200×). **A.** Oocyte secured by the holding pipette with the polar body positioned at 12 o'clock. **B.** Entry of the beveled micropipette through the zona pellucida. **C.** Aspiration of the polar body into the micropipette. **D.** Polar body removal complete. Polar body is visible in the micropipette.[1]

the follicle with a pH stable medium. Approximately 3 cc of PBS are injected into the follicle and aspirated, and the fluid is checked for the presence of the oocyte.

Phosphate buffered saline is prepared using a 1000-ml Nalgene receiver flask. Approximately 900 ml of HPLC grade water is added to antibiotics as for Ham's F-10 medium. For allergic patients, the antibiotics may be omitted. To this, 0.1 g of calcium chloride ($CaCl_2$, prepackaged) is added and mixed until dissolved. It is important to add the $CaCl_2$ prior to the PBS, otherwise the formation of intermediate salts will occur, rendering the solution unusable. Finally, the prepackaged PBS (9.6 g) is added and mixed until dissolved, and the volume is brought to 1000 ml. As with Ham's F-10, the osmolarity of the solution must be adjusted to within 278–282 mOsm. Usually the initial osmolarity is between 280 and 290 mOsm and may not

[1] This procedure is also shown on the cover: fluorescence, used for demonstration purposes, should not be applied in clinical practice to avoid possible damage to genetic material.

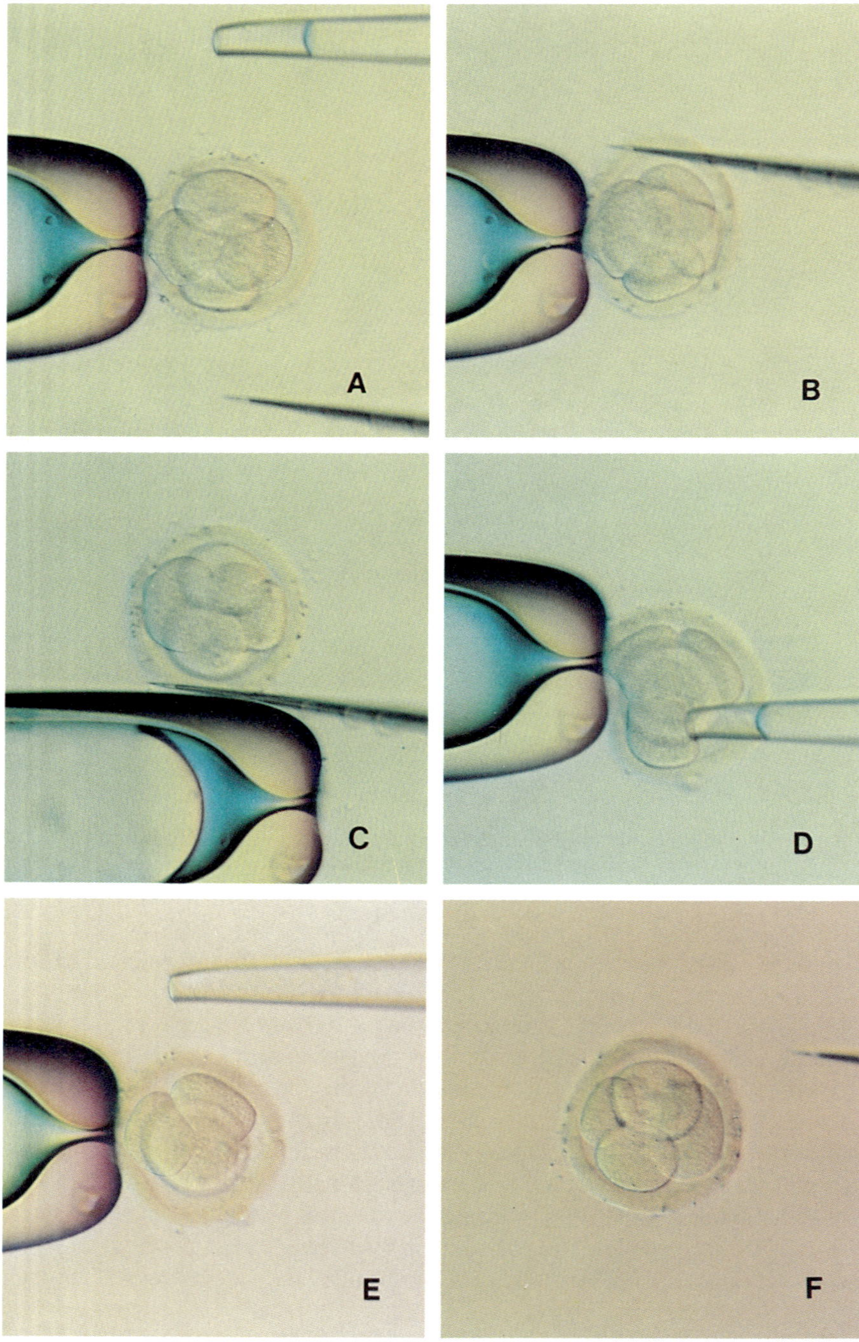
A
B
C
D
E
F

require adjustment at all. After the appropriate osmolarity has been reached, the solution is sterile filtered and aliquoted into 200-ml culture flasks until needed. The day before the scheduled aspiration, heparin (10 IU/ml, for preparation see below) is added to a 200-ml flask of PBS to inhibit the clotting of bloody follicular flushes which can make it difficult to visualize the oocyte. The flask of PBS with heparin is placed in a small incubator set at 37°C to warm overnight.

To prepare heparin (10 IU/ml), a 100,000 unit bottle of Heparin is dissolved in 250 ml of HPLC grade water and sterile filtered through a 0.2-micron filter. This is aliquoted into 50-ml culture flasks and stored at 0–5°C until needed. Exactly 5 ml of heparin is added to 200 ml of PBS to obtain a concentration of 10 IU/ml.
Reagents required for culture and micromanipulation are listed in Table II.

Polar Body Removal

Preparation for PGD prior to the retrieval of the oocytes is imperative. All microtools are constructed in advance with the number of aspirating pipettes slightly exceeding the number of oocytes expected (based on the estradiol level and ultrasound results the day HCG is given). The microtools are stored in sterile petri dishes (150 × 15 mm) until needed.

Several days prior to retrieval of the oocytes, the media and sterile equilibrated paraffin oil which will be used during micromanipulation must be prepared, and a sample of each must be given to the DNA laboratory for testing. All solutions used in conjunction with the biopsy must be free of DNA! If it is determined that there is DNA contamination, there must be a sufficient amount of time to submit new solutions for testing. For PBR the medium is supplemented with 0.1 molar sucrose to allow for ooplasm shrinkage thus decreasing the chance of damage and polyspermy (J. Cohen, personal communication). The medium is kept under sterile conditions at 5°C until it is needed.

As with routine IVF procedures, on the day before oocyte retrieval, 4-well culture dishes (one dish for each oocyte) containing IVF medium which is covered with sterile equilibrated paraffin oil are placed in the incubator overnight. At the same time, micromanipulation dishes are prepared with IVF medium and sucrose, using the lids from 35 × 10 mm Petri dishes. Two drops of medium are placed on the inside of the lid and flooded with the DNA-free oil tested previously. The number of dishes needed would again slightly exceed the number of oocytes expected. It is important to prepare

Figure 9 Biopsy of a triploid embryo (magnification 200×). **A.** Embryo is secured by the holding pipette and all microtools are aligned in the same focal plane. **B.** Partial zona dissection. The PZD needle is passed through the zona pellucida. **C.** Sawing of the zona pellucida. The PZD needle is placed over the holding pipette, gently pressed down onto the holding pipette, and with a sawing motion the slit is completed. **D.** Entry of the blunt-end micropipette into the embryo. **E.** The biopsy is complete and the blastomere is visible in the micropipette. **F.** Triploid embryo after biopsy.

one micromanipulation dish per oocyte to reduce the chance of contamination from the operator(s). These dishes are placed inside a larger 150 × 15 mm sterile Petri dish, which is placed in the incubator to equilibrate. The use of the 35 × 10 mm lids allows easy transport of oocytes on and off the microscope stage, without having to realign the holding pipette for each manipulation.

To perform PBR, a holding pipette with an inner diameter of 15–30 μm is filled with light paraffin oil and connected to the hydraulic system using the micropipette holder. The beveled pipette with an inner diameter of approximately 15–18 μm is filled with silicone oil (12,500 centistokes) before it is attached to its hydraulic system with a micropipette holder. Before each micromanipulation, it is necessary to place an empty Petri dish on the microscope stage to avoid leakage of oil from the pipettes to the objectives and to align the instruments in such a way that they are parallel to the microscope stage. Once aligned, the instruments are raised and a micromanipulation dish containing one oocyte is placed on the stage. The instruments are then lowered into the dish, excess oil is removed from the outer surface of the pipettes and a small amount of medium is aspirated into the beveled pipette. Once the oocyte has been secured by the holding pipette using gentle suction, the oocyte can be oriented so that the first polar body is visualized at 12 o'clock, utilizing the beveled micropipette (Fig. 8A). It is also important that the outer surface of the zona pellucida be free of corona cells at the point of entry in order to avoid contamination of the micropipette with maternal DNA. Once the polar body and zona pellucida are in focus, the beveled micropipette is passed through the zona to the polar body (Fig. 8B and 8C). Gentle suction is applied to aspirate the polar body into the micropipette, and pressure from the hydraulic system is equilibrated before exiting from the cell to avoid damage to the oocyte. If the polar body is still attached to the ooplasm, further incubation is required for complete detachment. The beveled micropipette containing the polar body (Fig. 8D) is lifted out of the dish and is handed to an assistant wearing gloves. Special attention is required so as not to disconnect the micropipette from the hydraulic system. In addition to sterile attire, gloves must be worn by IVF laboratory technicians to avoid contamination from operator DNA. The assistant carefully lowers the tip of the micropipette into a microcentrifuge tube containing HPLC grade acrodisc filtered water. A binocular magnifier (Stoelting, #51578) may be used to better visualize the tip as it descends into the water; this helps to avoid breaking the tip along the side of the tube. Once in the water, the polar body is expelled by several rotations of the micrometer (which is connected to the microsyringe). Before removing the micropipette, the tip is crushed on the bottom of the microcentrifuge tube to insure that the polar body is left in the water, if it happens to be stuck along the side of the micropipette.

The oocyte is released from the holding pipette, washed in IVF culture medium to remove sucrose, and transferred back to its original dish to await insemination.

Approximately 30 to 60 minutes after micromanipulation, oocytes are inseminated with 100,000 motile sperm and placed in the incubator for the night.

The next morning fertilization is determined by pronuclear formation and the presence of the second polar body.

After an additional 24 hours in culture, embryos are examined for cleavage (they have usually reached the 2 to 4-cell stage by then). At this time any diploid embryos (not to exceed three) that are considered to be unaffected by the particular disease can be transferred back to the patient's uterus with the hope of achieving a pregnancy. Any excess unaffected embryos are cryopreserved for transfer in subsequent cycles. Embryos which are considered to be affected, heterozygous, or whose diagnosis is inconclusive will be kept in culture to await blastomere biopsy.

Blastomere Biopsy

Embryo biopsy can be performed as soon as the embryo reaches the 3-cell stage, but it is preferable to biopsy at a later stage (before compaction) when a loss of one blastomere will cause less of a reduction in cell number (Hogan et al., 1986; Handyside et al., 1990).

A few ways in which blastomere biopsy can be accomplished are: zona drilling using an acid Tyrode's solution and a blunt-end micropipette (Handyside et al., 1990); partial zona dissection in which a microneedle is passed through an area of the zona pellucida to create an opening and a blunt-end micropipette is inserted; or entry and removal using a beveled micropipette. The latter only requires a single beveled micropipette. We are currently using the last two methods for this procedure, since the use of an acid Tyrode's solution may acidify the remaining blastomeres (Depypere et al., 1990).

The microtools for blastomere biopsy using a beveled micropipette are the same as for PBR, although it is preferable to use a beveled pipette with a larger diameter (18–25 mcm). Micromanipulation dishes are prepared in the same way as for PBR, using IVF medium without sucrose; the dishes are also previously analyzed for DNA contamination. During aspiration the cell membrane usually breaks; therefore, it is better to choose a blastomere with a clearly visible nucleus so that its aspiration into the pipette can be controlled and the chance of losing genetic material is reduced. Orientation of the embryo so that the blastomere nucleus and zona pellucida are in focus can be accomplished using the beveled pipette. It is very critical to avoid aspiration of any sperm attached to the zona pellucida when positioning or entering the embryo. Once aspirated into the micropipette, the blastomere nucleus is expelled into the microcentrifuge tube as in PBR.

In order to remove an intact blastomere for cytogenetic or molecular analysis, a larger opening is required. Two microtools are used for this purpose: a microneedle to create the opening in the zona, and a blunt-end micropipette to remove the blastomere. The blunt-end micropipette, with an inner diameter of 25–35 μm is filled with silicone oil of high viscosity (60,000 centistokes) in order to maintain good control despite the large diameter of the pipette. Both microtools are aligned in the same focal plane, side by side, using a double pipette holder (Narishige #HMD-2)(Fig. 9A). First, the microneedle is used for PZD (Fig. 9B and 9C). Once the slit is made in the zona, the embryo is oriented in such a way that the slit is visible around 3 o'clock. Second, the blunt-end micropipette is allowed to enter through the slit, and to remove the blastomere with suction created by the microsyringe (Fig. 9D, 9E, and 9F). The drawback of this method is that early "hatching" of uncompacted blastomeres can occur when the pressure from cleaving cells is exerted near the opening. Therefore, it is preferable to create a small slit in the zona during PZD.

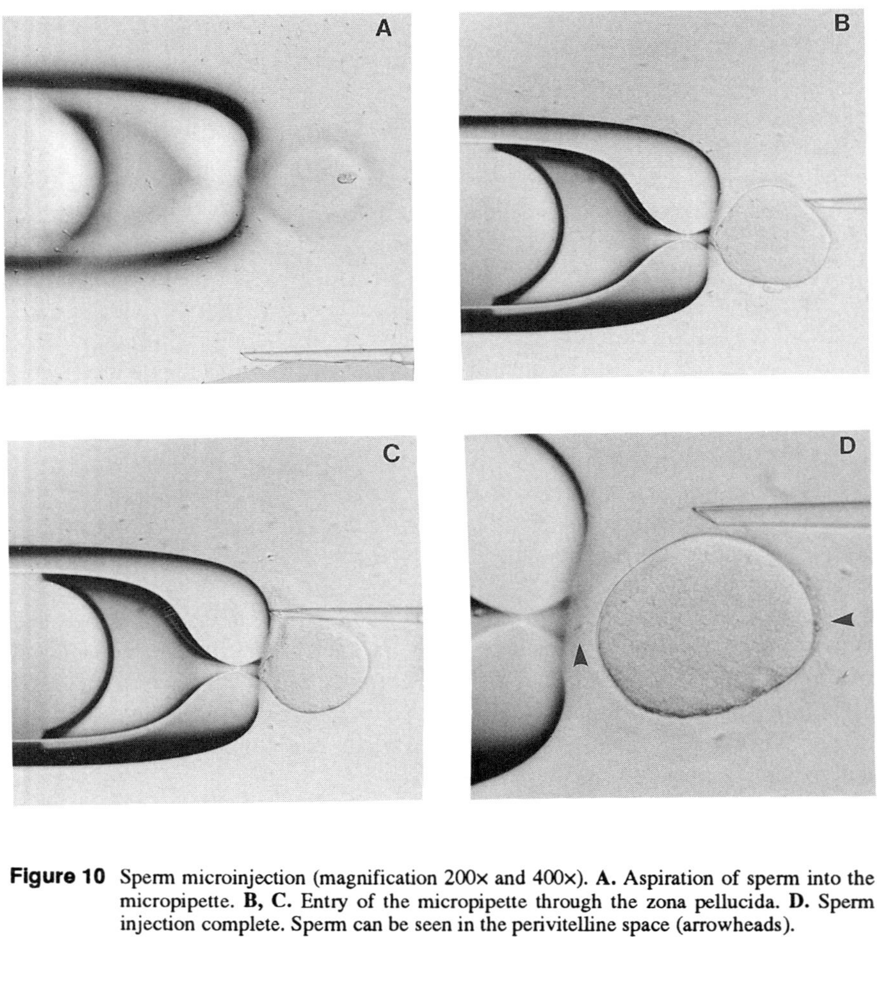

Figure 10 Sperm microinjection (magnification 200× and 400×). **A.** Aspiration of sperm into the micropipette. **B, C.** Entry of the micropipette through the zona pellucida. **D.** Sperm injection complete. Sperm can be seen in the perivitelline space (arrowheads).

Blastocyst Biopsy

When an embryo develops to an expanded blastocyst, a few trophectoderm cells can be taken for genetic analysis (Summers et al., 1988).

The procedure is performed in two steps:

1. Using the same set up as for PZD, the zona is dissected above the trophectoderm cells opposite the inner cell mass. After PZD, the blastocyst is placed in culture until it begins to hatch through the opening made in the zona.
2. Using a microneedle, herniated trophectoderm cells are pressed to the bottom of the Petri dish. While moving the needle back and forth, assurance is made that the "neck" of the herniated blastocyst is sealed. The herniated piece is cut away by a razor blade attached to a metal arm held by the micromanipulator. This procedure can also be performed under a dissecting microscope by hand using a scalpel blade (N15). The biopsied cells are transferred into a microcentrifuge tube for genetic analysis using a sterile Pasteur pipette.

Assisted Fertilization Techniques and Other Relevant Micromanipulations

Micromanipulation of oocytes to enhance fertilization is performed in cases where there is a male factor present and fertilization has failed to occur during a routine IVF procedure. The procedure performed depends on the semen parameters (especially the number of motile sperm per ml, rate of forward progression, and morphology). Before micromanipulation, all oocytes are liberated from their cumulus masses using hyaluronidase as described previously. If normal-appearing sperm with forward progressive movement are seen in the final concentration of sperm after processing, PZD is performed. In cases where the number of sperm is extremely low ($<1 \times 10^5$ per ml), forward progression is extremely poor (Grade 1), or if the percentage of normal forms is very low (<20%), microinjection into the perivitelline space or subzonal insemination is performed.

To perform sperm microinjection, the diameter of the beveled pipette should be 6–10 μm. In most cases unless the grade of movement is extremely poor, the micropipette is filled with silicone oil (12,500 centistokes) for quick control when aspirating sperm into the micropipette. A small drop of IVF medium containing sperm is placed in a micromanipulation dish and covered with equilibrated paraffin oil as for other micromanipulation procedures. Several oocytes can be placed in the single drop, providing the operator is proficient; otherwise it may be prudent to transfer the oocytes one at a time. An oocyte is secured by the holding pipette using gentle suction from the microsyringe. From one to several sperm (depending upon morphology) are aspirated into the micropipette using a quick twist of the micrometer attached to the microsyringe. It is easier to pick up sperm along the edge of the drop of medium one is working in, where the most motile sperm are usually found (Fig. 10A). Once the sperm are in the micropipette, it is essential to equilibrate the pressure so there is no flow of medium into or out of the micropipette. Sperm should be aspirated into the micropipette, tail first, to facilitate swimming out on their own into the perivitelline space. Once the sperm have been aspirated, the oocyte must be brought back into focus and the zona pellucida must be punctured before the sperm reach the tip of the pipette (Fig. 10B, 10C, and 10D). This must be done quickly or the sperm will escape out into the medium. The oocytes are returned to the incubator for a minimum of 6 hours before they can be examined for the presence of pronuclei.

Our experience has shown that there is an increase in polyspermy when this procedure is performed. However, decreasing the number of injected sperm or injecting only one sperm (especially when there are <20% normal forms present) may reduce the chance of fertilization even further. Perhaps the microinjection of acrosome reacted sperm which can be achieved artificially may increase the efficieny of this procedure.

Pronucleus Removal

For research purposes, it might be necessary to transform a triploid zygote into a diploid state by microsurgical removal of the extra pronucleus. The beveled needle used for enucleation should be 18–20 μm in diameter, flame-polished, and siliconized.

Ten to 15 minutes before the beginning of micromanipulation, the zygote is placed in a medium containing 1–2 micrograms per milliliter of cytochalasin B, and enucleation is performed in the same medium. The main principle is that the plasma membrane of the zygote is not punctured, i.e., the pronucleus is removed as a karyoplast. This method, proposed by McGrath and Solter (1983), still remains the only reliable approach to zygote enucleation. However, no method exists for distinguishing male and female pronuclei, so that there is the risk that the female pronucleus may be removed, leaving both male pronuclei in the zygote. As such an androgenetic embryo may result in a hydatid mole, restored diploidy does not make it acceptable for transfer.

References

Depypere HT, Leybaert L, Dhont M, de Hemptinne A, Vandekerckhove D (1990): The intracytoplasmatic pH change during zona drilling of mouse oocytes. Hum Reprod 5(Suppl):6–7.

Handyside AH, Kontogianni EH, Hardy K, Winston RML (1990): Pregnancies from biopsied human preimplantation embryos sexed by Y-specific DNA amplification. Nature 344:768–770.

Hogan B, Constantini F, Lacy E (1986): "Manipulating the mouse embryo. A Laboratory Manual," New York: Cold Spring Harbor Laboratory.

Malter HE, Cohen J (1989): Partial zona dissection of the human oocyte: A nontraumatic method using micromanipulation to assist zona pellucida penetration. Fertil Steril 51:139.

McGrath J, Solter D (1983): Nuclear transplantation in the mouse embryo by microsurgery and cell function. Science 220:1300–1319.

Summers PM, Campbell JM, Miller MW (1988): Normal in vivo development of marmoset monkey embryos after trophectoderm biopsy. Hum Reprod 3:389–393.

CHAPTER 7

DNA Analysis of Polar Bodies and Preembryos

Charles M. Strom and Svetlana Rechitsky

In preimplantation genetic analysis, diagnosis must be accomplished within 72 hours of oocyte harvest in order to transfer preembryos during the same cycle. This precludes freezing of the embryos and the resultant reduction of the implantation rate (Handyside et al., 1989, 1990; Verlinsky et al., 1990a, 1990b). The advent of the polymerase chain reaction (PCR) enables genetic diagnosis to be performed on DNA from a single cell in less than 72 hours (Li et al., 1988; Handyside et al., 1989; Coutelle et al., 1989; Strom et al., 1990; Verlinsky et al., 1990b). PCR is a method of amplifying specific DNA sequences. Specific oligonucleotide primers are synthesized complimentary to genetic sequences bracketing the sequence to be amplified. These primers are designed in opposite orientations on complimentary strands of DNA to allow the PCR to logarithmically amplify the internal sequences (Fig. 1).

The PCR reaction is able to amplify DNA from single sperm, polar bodies, blastomeres, amniocytes, and fibroblasts.

Several important systems must be optimized to reliably amplify DNA from single cells. These include elimination and/or prevention of contamination with extraneous DNA sequences, and optimization of cell lysis conditions, primer design, PCR specificity, and appropriate internal controls. Even with these precautions, PCR analysis could potentially lead to a misdiagnosis if one of the two alleles of a heterozygous cell failed to amplify, a process we describe as allele-specific PCR failure. This chapter will describe PCR optimization for DNA analysis of single cells which forms the basis of preimplantation genetic analysis. The list of equipment and reagents needed in DNA analysis of polar bodies and preembryos is presented in Tables I and II.

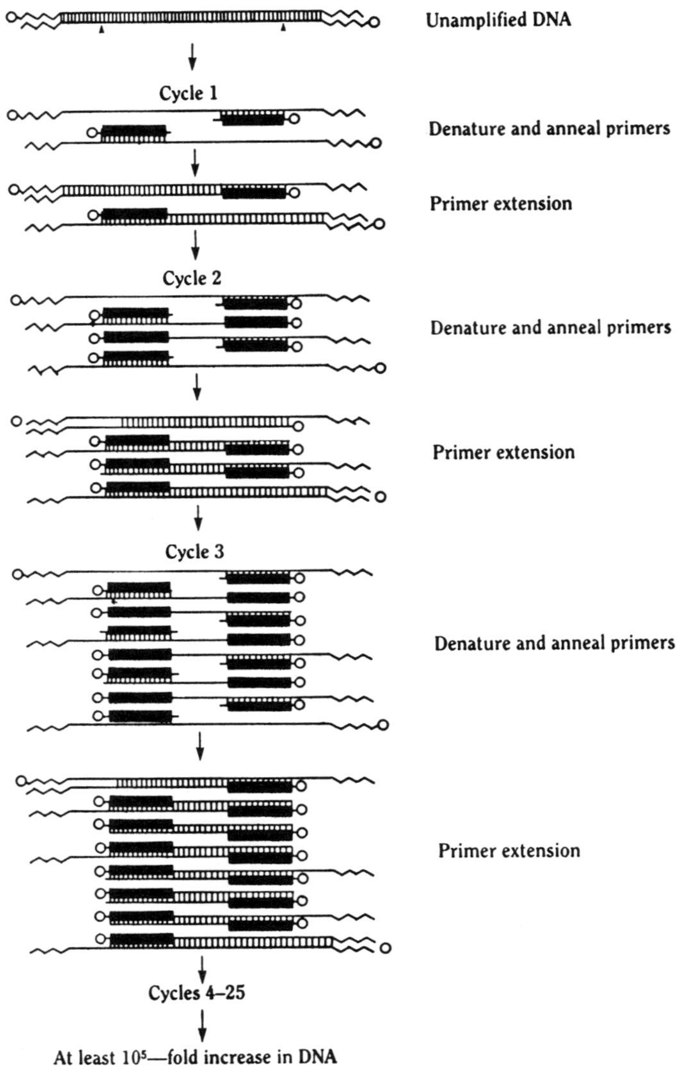

Figure 1 Polymerase chain reaction (Perkin Elmer Cetus, 1990).

Optimization of PCR for Single Cells

Cell Lysis

Polar bodies and blastomeres are easier to lyse than somatic cells such as amniocytes and fibroblasts. Several methods of cell lysis for single cells can be used: proteinase K treatment, freeze-thaw in PCR buffer, and freeze-thaw in distilled water. The best PCR results are obtained using the following protocol. The single cell is obtained by micromanipulation, placed into distilled water at room temperature for at least 10 minutes and frozen at -80°C for at least 20 minutes. Frozen samples can be stored for several days at this temperature without a significant decline in PCR amplification. Following the freezing, the samples are incubated at 99°C for 15 minutes prior to the addition of PCR buffer and the beginning of "hot start" PCR. (See following section regarding "hot start" PCR.)

We have shown that the potassium hydroxide lysis technique described by Li et al. (1991) for single sperm is the optimal method of single cell lysis for preimplantation analysis.

Reaction Conditions

Reaction conditions must be individually optimized for each primer set and PCR reaction. All parameters must be adjusted in order to obtain optimal results. As a general rule, the most stringent reaction conditions consistent with successful amplification should be used for each case. Tables III and IV summarize the reaction conditions for each of the primer sets currently used in our laboratory.

1. The *magnesium concentration* must be separately adjusted for each primer set. Therefore, PCR buffers without Mg should be used so that varying amounts of Mg can be added to each reaction.
2. *Optimization of Glycerol and formamide concentration* is essential as they increase the specificity of the reaction by increasing the hybridization stringency (Sarkar et al., 1990; Pomp and Medrano, 1991). In addition, glycerol may stabilize the Taq polymerase and allow better efficiency of polymerization when extended cycles of PCR are used.
3. We have found that two-temperature PCR (*"turbo PCR"*) is just as effective as the standard three-step PCR for single-cell amplification. The use of two-temperature PCR decreases cycle times significantly and allows for more rapid completion of PCR, a crucial element in preimplantation diagnosis. For most reactions, 20 seconds at 95°C in a Perkin-Elmer Cetus thermal cycler model 9600 is sufficient for melting. The time for the annealing polymerization can be varied. The initial 10 cycles usually require 1 minute at the annealing temperature, and shorter times (30 sec) can be used for later cycles. Using these

Table I Required Materials and Reagents for Preimplantation DNA Analysis

Item		Source
Ampli Taq DNA polymerase,250 units		Perkin Elmer Cetus, N801-0060
GeneAmp dNTPs(10mM dATP, 10mM dCTP, 10mM dTTP, 10mM dGTP)		Perkin Elmer Cetus, N808-0007
DNA size marker D8397		Perkin Elmer Cetus, N930-2106
DNA marker: 123 base-pair ladder		Gibco BRL
Mineral oil		Perkin Elmer Cetus, N0186-2302
Restricted enzyme Mse-I		New England Biolabs, #525
HPLC water chromatography grade		Mallinckrodt Inc. Scientific Products, 6795-1NY
Ethidium bromide tablets		Bio-Rad, 161-0430
Bromphenol blue		Bio-Rad, 161-0404
Ammonium persulfate		Bio-Rad, 161-0700
TEMED (N,N,N',N'-Tetramethylethylenediamine)		Bio-Rad, 161-0800
Acrylamide		Bibco,BRL 5512 UA
N,N^1-methylenebisacrylamide		BRL 5516 UA
Sucrose		BRL 5503 UA
Potassium chloride		Fisher, P-217
TRIS HCl		Fisher Biotech, BP152-500
Boric acid		Fisher Biotech, BP168-500
Gelatin		Sigma, N G2500
Magnesium chloride		J.T. Baker Chemical Co., 2444-1
EDTA (Ethylenediaminetetraacetic acid)		J.T. Baker Chemical Co., 8993-1
Ammonium hydroxide		Fisher, A669-500
For allele-specific hybridization		
Denaturing solution		0.4M NaOH, 25mM Na_2EDTA
20 × SSPE	3.6M NaCl 20mM NaH_2PO_4 20mM Na_2 EDTA	pH 7.4 (adjust with NaOH pellet)
10% SDS		
100 × Denhardt's solution		2% Ficoll 400 (Sigma) 2% PVP - 360 (Sigma) 2% BSA (Pentax FractionV) (Gibco BRL)
Prehybridization solution		5 × SSPE 5 × Denhardt's solution 0.5% SDS (Fisher) 0.1 mg/ml herring sperm (Boehringer Mannheim)

(Continued)

Table I Required Materials and Reagents for Preimplantation DNA Analysis (Continued)

Wash solution	2 × SSPE 0.1% SDS

For end-labeling

Allele-specific oligonucleotides (ASO)
T4 polynucleotide kinase with recommended buffer (Gibco BRL)
Biogel P4 in distilled H_2O (Bio-Rad)
Select - D columns (5' - 3') (5 Prime-3 Prime Inc.)

Cloned Taq DNA polymerase	5 units/μl	(AmpliTaq; Perkin-Elmer Cetus)
10× reaction buffer	100 mM TRIS HCl (pH 8.3) 500 mM KCl	

Stock is made up in HPLC water, autoclaved, millipore filtered, aliquoted and stored at -20°C.

10×dNTPs	2.0mM of each of four dNTPs (Perkin-Elmer Cetus). Stock is aliquoted and stored at -20°C, thawed only for immediate use.
25mM mgCL$_2$	

Oligonucleotides

Oligonucleotides were synthesized on an Applied Biosystem 381-A DNA Synthesizer and eluted from the column in ammonium hydroxide solution (3–5 times), incubated overnight at 55°C, vacuum dried in speed vac concentrator.

Pellet was resuspended in 1ml of HPLC H_20 and optical density was measured using quartz currettes and a spectrophotometer with UV light source.

Oligos were diluted to 10μM.

Molarities calculated as:

363(#of Gs) + 323 (#of Cs) + 347 (#of As) + 322 (#of Ts) =gram grams/mole

Reaction mix (for 100μl reaction)

10× reaction buffer	10.0 μl
10× dNTPs	5.0 μl
Taq polymerase	1 unit (0.2 mcl) μM
Upstream primer	0.1 - 0.5 μM
Downstream primer	0.1 - 0.5 μM
50% glycerol	3 - 5 μl
or	
100% formamide	1 - 2 μl
H_20	to 100 μl

(Continued)

Table I Required Materials and Reagents for Preimplantation DNA Analysis (Continued)

For Electrophoresis		
Bromphenol blue dye:	50% sucrose 0.1m EDTA (pH 7.0) 0.05% Bromphenol blue dye	
Ethidium bromide:5mg/mcl in distilled H_20	Use 0.5 mcL/ml	
Electrophoresis buffer: 10×TBE (pH8.3)	1M TRIS HCl 1M Boric acid 20mM EDTA	
40% Bisacrylamide:	Acrylamide 38% N,N^1-methylene bisacrylamide 2%	
Acrylamide gel:	(6ml per 1 gel)	
	8%	12%
40% Bisacrylamide	1.2	1.8
10×TBE	0.6	0.6
10% Ammonium persulfate	0.075	0.075
TEMED	0.005	0.005
H_20	4.2	3.6

Abbreviations: PVP-360 = polyvinilpyrrolidone-360, BSA = bovine serum albumin, SDS = sodium dodecye sulfate.

guidelines it is usually possible to complete single-cell PCR amplifications in approximately 2 hours.

4. *Hot start PCR* involves withholding one or more of the required reagents of the PCR mix until the mixture is heated to at least 72°C. This prevents nonspecific annealing of primers and subsequent chain elongation of spurious DNA sequences in the first cycle of PCR (Faloona et al., 1990). The optimum method of "hot start" PCR for single cells is the following: heat the sample to 99°C in distilled water, add the PCR buffer without primers and Taq polymerase, heat to 72°C, and then add the samples with the Taq polymerase and primers in the thermal cycler, and begin the first PCR immediately.

Primer Design and Nested Amplification

Nested amplification significantly increases the efficiency of amplification of DNA from single cells (Mullis and Faloona, 1987; Li et al., 1991). It involves performing 20 cycles of PCR with one set of primers (outside primers), followed by removing of an aliquot of this reaction and adding it to a new reaction mixture that contains a primer, or primers, whose sequence is located between the two initial primers [inside primer(s)]. We have found that the best results are obtained by using lower stringency in the initial and higher stringency in the nested, reaction. Also, using a single inside nested primer (heminesting), with the appropriate original outside primer, is as efficient as using two inside primers for the second reaction (full nesting).

The use of nested primers has several advantages over simple PCR. In our laboratory it has increased the efficiency of single-cell PCR from 70% or 80% of single cells analyzed to more than 90%. In addition, nested PCR creates more PCR product than simple PCR and allows more manipulations to be carried out to optimize genotype analysis. An unexpected benefit of nested PCR is that problems arising from contamination with extraneous DNA sequences, such as in delta-F508 mutational analysis, are reduced dramatically. An explanation of this phenomenon is not immediately apparent. Perhaps intermittent contamination of reagents with synthetic DNA occurs, which lacks complimentarity to all four primers. Another possibility is that nested primer reactions tend to amplify larger fragments of DNA, and contamination with smaller fragments may not lead to successful amplification of the contaminating sequences. Further investigation will be necessary to determine if this reduction in detection of DNA contamination will be observed for other nested PCR reactions.

Eliminating and Preventing DNA Contamination

The well-described methods to avoid "carry-over" in the PCR reaction are inadequate to prevent contamination in single-cell PCR. It is important that all reagents including those used in the embryology laboratory, must be tested for DNA contamination prior to every preimplantation genetic diagnosis (PGD), since we have found that even in vitro fertilization (IVF) water, immersion oil, growth media, and human serum can become contaminated with extraneous DNA. To avoid the possibility of contamination it is essential to have separate preimplantation reagents in the embryology laboratory whose bottles are never touched without gloves. Usual sterile technique is not sufficient to avoid DNA contamination. For example, it is perfectly acceptable to handle micropipettes with bare hands while making microtools with respect to sterility; however, this can easily lead to contamination of the pipette with DNA sequences. Similarly, standard sterile techniques of handling bottles containing immersion oil and growth media with bare hands and flaming the neck of the bottles following their use are unacceptable for PGD.

In addition to using positive displacement pipettes and laminar flow hoods, gloves are worn at all times. A separate laboratory designated for PGD is advisable in which

Table II Required Equipment for Preimplantation DNA Analysis

Laminar flow (biological) biosafety cabinet	Edgegard Hood (Eg-3252)
Cetus Thermal Cycler	Perkin Elmer Cetus
Microfuge™ 12	Beckman
Freezer Revco (-80°C)	
Refrigerator (2–8°C)	
Freezer (-20°C)	
UV transilluminator C-62	Ultra-violet Products, Inc.
Camera FCR-10	Fotodyne Inc.
Polaroid film type 667	
Gel apparatus—mini-protean II	
dual slab cell	Bio-Rad, 165-2940
Electrophoresis power supply	Bio-Rad, model 100/200
pH meter	Fisher, model 955
Positive displacement pipettors	Rainin Instrument Co., micromen M-25, M-50, M-250
Pipettors, adjustable to deliver 1-1000 ml	Rainin Instrument Co., Gilson P-20, P-200, P-1000
Serological pipets	Fisher, #13-678-3114 disposable (5ml)
Serological pipets	Fisher, #13-676-10J disposable (10 ml)
Polycarbonate microcentrifuge tube opener	USA Scientific Plastics USA, 050
Microcentrifuge tube, flat cap (1.5 ml)	USA Scientific Plastics USA, 505-FT
Microcentrifuge tube, flat cap (0.5 ml)	USA Scientific Plastics USA, 502
50-Place (5×10) polypropylene storage box	USA Scientific Plastics, PB50-V
Microcentrifuge tube racks	Nalgene Company, #5973-0315
Transfer pipets	USA Scientific Plastics USA, 304
DNA synthesizer	Applied Biosystem, 381-A DNA synthesizer
Speed-vac concentrator	Savant
Refrigerated condensation trap	Savant
Cameo IIS 0.22-mm filter unit	MSI
Vortex—Genie 2	Scientific Industries
Slot blot apparatus	Bio-Rad
Minihybridization oven	Vanegard International
GM-counter	Ludlum Inc.
The belly dancer/hybridization water bath	Stovall Life Science Inc.

(Continued)

Table II Required Equipment for Preimplantation DNA Analysis *(Continued)*

Nylon membrane positively charged	Boehringer Mannheim
Laboratory glassware—including beakers, graduated cylinders,Erlenmeyer flasks.	
Disposables—gloves, lab wipes, Parafilm laboratory films, waterproof marking pen, UV goggles, Syringes	

no tubes containing PCR products are ever opened. All reagents are placed in separate small aliquots, so that if contamination occurs, a new bottle can be used immediately.

However, despite precautions, intermittent contamination will occur. Under these circumstances the reagents must be decontaminated using one of the following techniques. If the sequence to be amplified contains a restriction site, restriction digestion can be performed, followed by heat inactivation of the restriction enzyme to eliminate all double-stranded DNA (Verlinsky et al., 1990; Strom et al., 1991). If contamination is from single-stranded DNA, restriction digestion will not successfully decontaminate the reagent. In this circumstance, PCR must be performed for 5 to 10 cycles in order to convert the single-stranded DNA into double-stranded DNA so that restriction digestion may be applied to successfully decontaminate the reagent.

Nonspecific forms of decontamination of PCR reagents by ultraviolet irradiation or psoralen treatment may be also used (Jinno et al., 1990; Sarkar and Sommer, 1990a, 1991). Ultraviolet radiation requires the use of thin-walled PCR tubes, and of both 254-nm and 300-nm light boxes, for a minimum of 10 minutes at each wavelength immediately prior to PCR. However, storage of irradiated products prior to PCR often results in the appearance of confusing nonspecific PCR bands in blanks and assays. As for psoralen treatment, it has not been found to be reliable for decontaminating single-cell PCR reagents.

Another of the difficulties in single-cell PCR is the phenomenon of pseudocontamination, when the blank lanes contain PCR products at, or near the expected band of the true sequence. Digestion of these PCR products with restriction enzymes known to have sites in the amplified region can demonstrate that these sequences are not the expected amplified sequence. Pseudocontamination can be eliminated by using nested primers, or increasing the stringency of the PCR reaction by lowering concentrations of dNTPs, Mg, or Taq polymerase.

In any event, it is imperative that any preimplantation diagnosis assay contain several control assays with no added cell or DNA, false biopsies, and fully reconstituted PCR mixtures in order to assure that there is no contamination with extraneous DNA sources. Positive controls, containing 100 pg of homozygous abnormal, homozygous normal, and heterozygous DNA, must also be included in each case.

Table III PGD by Single-Cell PCR Analysis: Primers and Reaction Conditions

Locus		Primer Sequence (5'–3')	$MgCl_2$ (mM)	Primer (mcM)	Temp. (°C)	Time (sec)	Number of cycles
Cystic fibrosis	Forward	GACTTCACTTCTAATGATGAT	2	0.1	92	20	10
trans-	outside						
membrane	Reverse	CTCTTCTAGTTGGCATGC	2	0.1	92	20	15
regulator	outside					45	30
(CFTR)					72	60	
Delta F-508	Forward	CAGTGGAAGAATTTCATTCTGTTCTCA	2	0.2	93	20	
mutation	inside				57	30	30
exon 10	reverse	GTTGGCATGCTTTGATGACGCTTC	2	0.2	70	45	
	inside	(Kerem et al., 1989)					
ß-Hexosam-	Forward	GTGTGGCGAGAGGATATTCCAGT	1.5	0.3	92	20	40
inidase A							
exon 11					64	60	
(Tay-Sach's							
disease)	Reverse	TTCAAATGCCAGGGGTTCCACTA	1.5	0.3			
		(Myerowitz and Costigan, 1988)					
Factor VIII	7.1	CACGAGCTCTCCATCTGAACATG	2	0.2	94	20	10
XbaI RFLP	Forward					60	60
(Hemophilia A)					94	20	
intron 22	7.10	GGGCTGCAGGGGGGGGGACAACAG	2	0.15	60	30	35
	Reverse	(Kogan et al., 1987)					

Factor VIII	7.1			0.2			
XbaI RFLP	7.10			0.2	94	20	45
Alphoid					55	90	
repeats of							
the human	Y1	ATGATAGAACGGAAATATG	2.5	0.5			
Y chromosome	Y2	AGTAGAATGCAAAGGGCTCC		0.5			
(simultaneous		(Wolfe et al., 1985)					
amplification)							
Alphoid	Y1			0.5			
repeats of	Y2		2.5	0.5	94	20	45
the human					64	30	
X chromosome	X1	AATCATCAAATGGAGATTTG		0.25	50	30	
(simultaneous	X2	GTTCAGCTCTGTGAGTGAAA		0.25	72	60	
amplification)		(Waye et al., 1985)					
Alpha-1-anti-	Forward	TCAGCCTTACAACGTGTCTCT		0.5			
trypsin			1.5		93	20	
(PI type Z)					53	45	45
	Reverse	GTTTGTTGAACTTGACCTCG		0.5	70	45	
		(Dermer and Johnson, 1988)					

Following 40–45 cycles of PCR, chain elongation was carried out by incubation at 72°C for 8–10 min.

Genotyping Polar Bodies and Blastomeres

Detection of PCR Products

We have employed three different techniques to analyze PCR products, depending on the mutation being analyzed. For the delta-F508 mutation in the cystic fibrosis transmembrane regulator (CFTR) and the insertion mutation in the hexosaminidase gene, we use the *heteroduplex detection method* (Rommens et al., 1990; Triggs-Raine and Gravel, 1990). In this technique the PCR products are mixed with PCR products from known homozygous normal and homozygous mutant alleles. After mixing the tubes are heated and then the DNA is allowed to reanneal, forming heteroduplexes. The DNA is electrophoresed through polyacrylamide gels and the bands are directly visualized on ethidium bromide stained gels. Figure 2 demonstrates a preconception

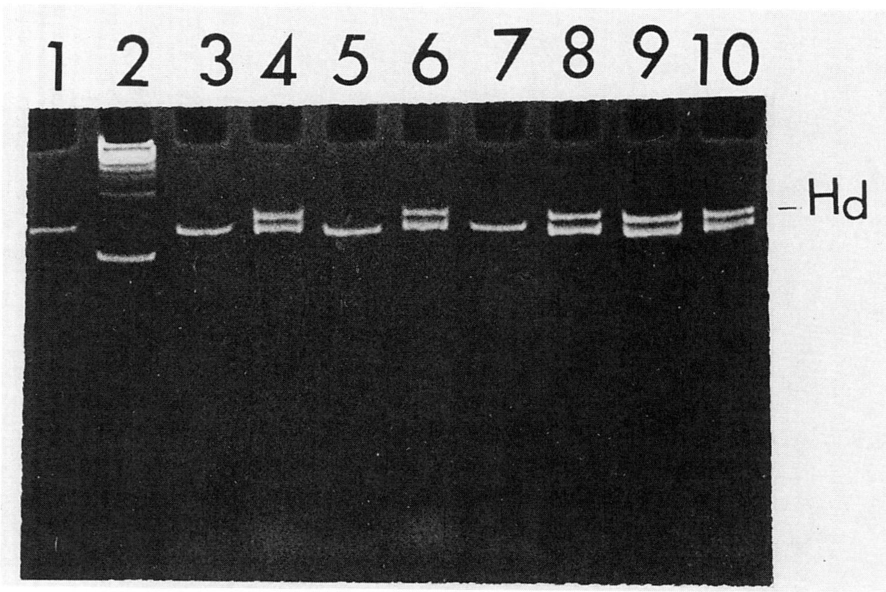

Figure 2 PCR analysis of DNA from the first polar body following PBR: nested amplification with cystic fibrosis primers flanking delta-F508 mutation site. **Lane 1.** Homozygous normal polar body DNA. **Lane 2.** Size markers 123 base pair ladder. **Lane 3.** Homozygous normal polar body DNA mixed with homozygous normal amplified DNA. **Lane 4.** Homozygous normal polar body DNA mixed with delta-F508 amplified DNA. **Lane 5.** Homozygous delta-F508 normal polar body DNA. **Lane 6.** Homozygous delta-F508 polar body DNA mixed with homozygous normal amplified DNA. **Lane 7.** Homozygous delta-F508 polar body DNA mixed with delta-F508 amplified DNA. **Lane 8.** Heterozygous polar body DNA. **Lane 9.** Heterozygous polar body DNA mixed with homozygous normal DNA. **Lane 10.** Heterozygous polar body DNA mixed with delta-F508 DNA.

Table IV Slot Blot Analysis of PCR Products from Polar Bodies, Blastomeres, and Single Somatic Cells: Allele-Specific Oligonucleotides and Reaction Conditions

Locus		Probe sequence (5'–3')	Hybridization temperature (°C)	Stringency washes	
				Time (min)	Temp (°C)
Cystic fibrosis transmembrane regulator (CFTR)	normal	CHCCAAAGATGATATTTTC	45	2 ×10 2 ×5	room temp 45
Delta-F508 mutation exon 10	mutant	AACACCA—ATGATATTTTCTT	45		
Factor VIII XbaI RFLP	7.3	GCGCATTTCT<u>A</u>GACTGTTG	50	2 ×10 2 ×5	room temp 52
intron 22 (hemophilia A)	7.4	GCGCATTTCT<u>G</u>GACTGTTG (Kogan et al., 1987)	50	2 ×10 2 ×5	room temp 54
Alpha-1-antitrypsin PI type Z	normal	TCCCTTTCT<u>C</u>GTCGATGGT	45	2 ×10 2 ×5	room temp 55
	mutant	TCCCTTTCT<u>T</u>GTCGATGGT	45	2 ×10	room temp
β-Hexosaminidase A exon 11	normal	GAACCGTATAT—CCTATGGC	40	2 ×10 2 ×5	room temp 48
(Tay-Sach's disease)	mutant	GAACCGTATAT<u>CTAT</u>CCTA (Myerowitz and Costigan, 1988)	40	2 ×10 2 ×5	room temp 52

diagnosis for the delta-F508 mutation using polar body removal. The polar body diagnoses are easily made by examining the gel.

Figure 3 represents a preconception genetic diagnosis for the insertion mutation of Tay-Sach's disease. Again, the heteroduplexes are easily seen and an unambiguous diagnosis is possible for two of the three polar bodies. PCR failure occurred in the third analysis.

A second method of genetic analysis following single-cell PCR is shown in Figure 4, which represents a preconception genetic diagnosis, following PBR, for the XbaI mutation in the factor VIII gene. In this analysis, restriction digestion of the PCR products is performed prior to electrophoresis, and the presence or absence of the site can be detected (Kogan et al., 1987, 1990). The analysis can be complicated by the amplifications of pseudogenes, but if high stringency is used, these extraneous bands can be minimized. However, even in the homozygous state for the presence of the site,

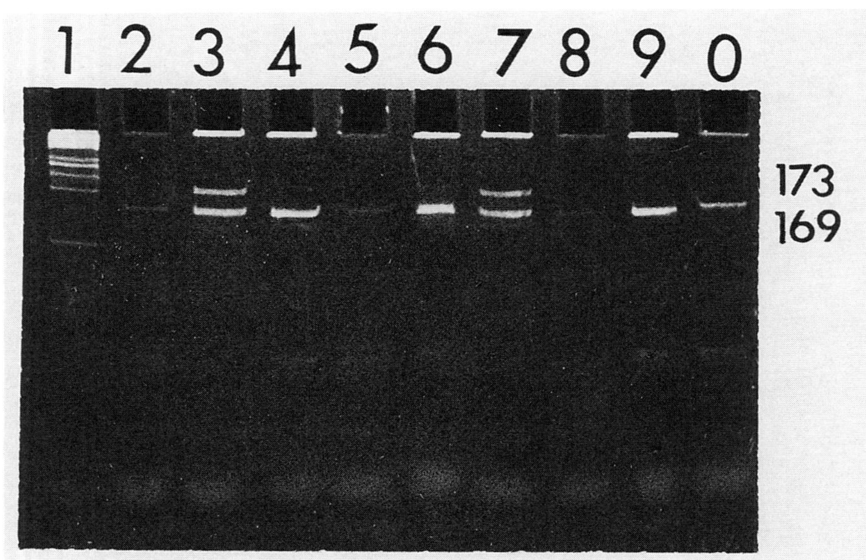

Figure 3 Genetic prediction of Tay-Sach's disease by polar body DNA amplification: heterozygosity for the exon 11 insertion allele, detected by the anomalous migration of normal/mutant heteroduplexes in nondenaturating 10% polyacrilamide gel. **Lane 1.** Size markers 123 base pair ladder. **Lane 2.** Homozygous abnormal polar body DNA. **Lane 3.** Homozygous abnormal polar body DNA mixed with amplified homozygous normal DNA. **Lane 4.** Homozygous abnormal polar body DNA mixed with amplified homozygous inserted DNA. **Lane 5.** Homozygous normal polar body DNA. **Lane 6.** Homozygous normal polar body DNA mixed with homozygous normal DNA. **Lane 7.** Homozygous normal polar body DNA mixed with homozygous inserted DNA. **Lane 8.** Failed amplification of polar body DNA. **Lane 9.** Failed amplification of polar body DNA mixed with homozygous normal DNA. **Lane 10.** Failed amplification of polar body DNA mixed with homozygous inserted DNA.

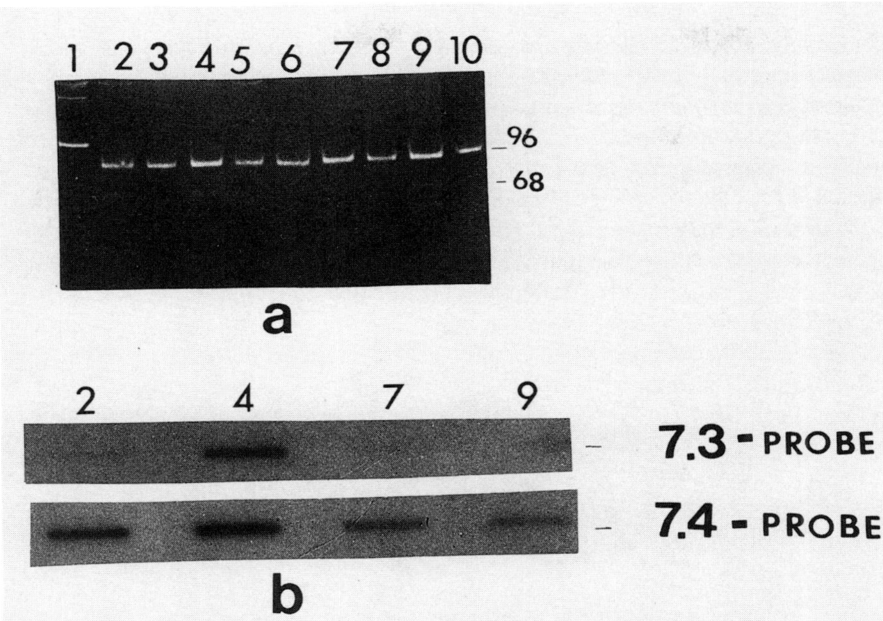

Figure 4 Preimplantation analysis of the XbaI polymorphism in amplified DNA from the first polar body (the hemophilia A mutation in this family was found to correspond to the presence of the XBaI digestion site in intron 22). **a.** PCR products from polar bodies in lanes 3,5,6,8, and 10 were not digested with XbaI enzyme, so corresponding oocytes were identified as being unaffected. The digestion site was found in amplified DNA from four polar bodies in lanes 2,4,7, and 9; this predicted that the corresponding oocytes were affected. **b.** Similar results are demonstrated by allele- specific hybridization with synthetic oligonucleotides probes: 7.3 corresponds to the presence of the XbaI RFLP site, and 7.4 designates the absence of the digestion site.

undigested material remains. Because of this potential source of error we simultaneously perform allele-specific hybridization analysis (described below) and only oocytes confirmed to be unaffected by both methods are transferred.

The third method of genetic analysis is allele-specific hybridization of duplicate-slot blot filters. This method is used for alpha-1-antitrypsin PI type ZZ deficiency, the Xba1 polymorphism, and retinitis pigmentosa, and can also be used for the delta-F508 mutation in the CFTR. Figure 4 shows a preconception analysis of the Xba1 restriction fragment length polymorphism (RFLP).

Allele-Specific PCR Failure

A potential problem when using PCR to analyze the DNA of a single cell for a single-copy gene is a failure to amplify one of the two alleles in a heterozygous individual, an event we have named allele-specific PCR failure. If the PCR fails completely (total PCR failure) no diagnosis will be possible and therefore no diagnostic error will be made. However, if allele-specific PCR failure occurs in a heterozygous cell, the cellular genotype will be mistakenly identified as homozygous rather than heterozygous (Navadi and Arnheim, 1991). A single cell will have two template strands for each of the two alleles (the sense and missense strand of each allele). If the DNA should become damaged for both alleles of the one sequence, leaving the complimentary gene intact, PCR analysis would amplify only one sequence and the cell would appear to be homozygous when, in fact, it is heterozygous.

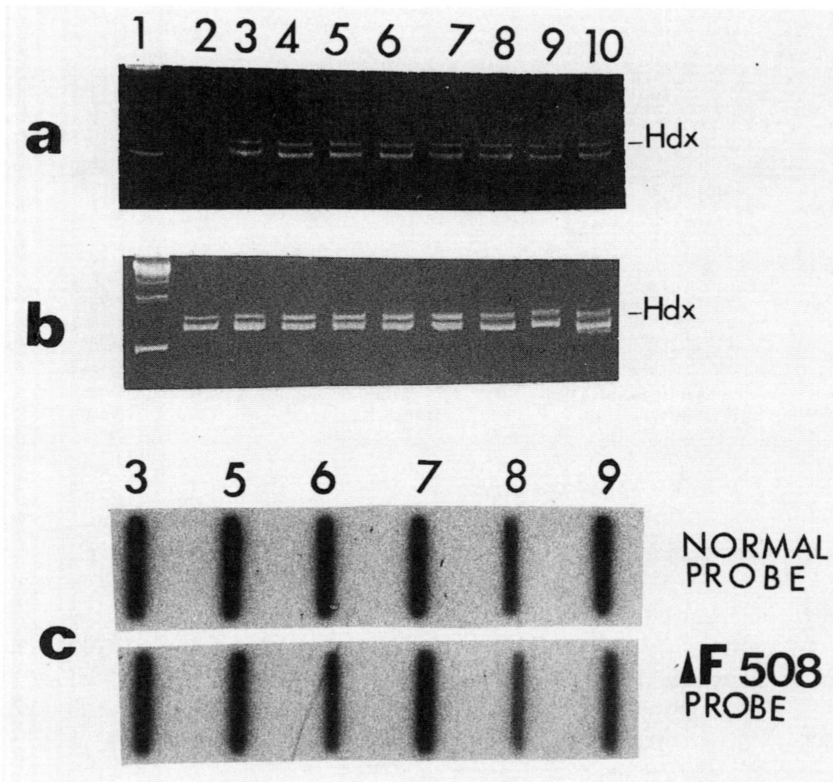

Figure 5 PCR analysis of single skin fibroblasts heterozygous for the delta-F508 mutation in the CFTR gene, showing no allele-specific PCR failure. **a.** 40 cycles of PCR with inside set of primers flanking exon 10 with three base pair deletion. **b.** Nested amplification. 25 cycles of PCR with outside set of primers and 30 cycles of amplification with inside set of primers (see Table II). (A heteroduplex between the normal and mutant sequences is detected as extra bands of slower mobility). **c.** Duplicate slot blots of PCR products hybridized with oligonucleotides specific to the normal and mutant allele.

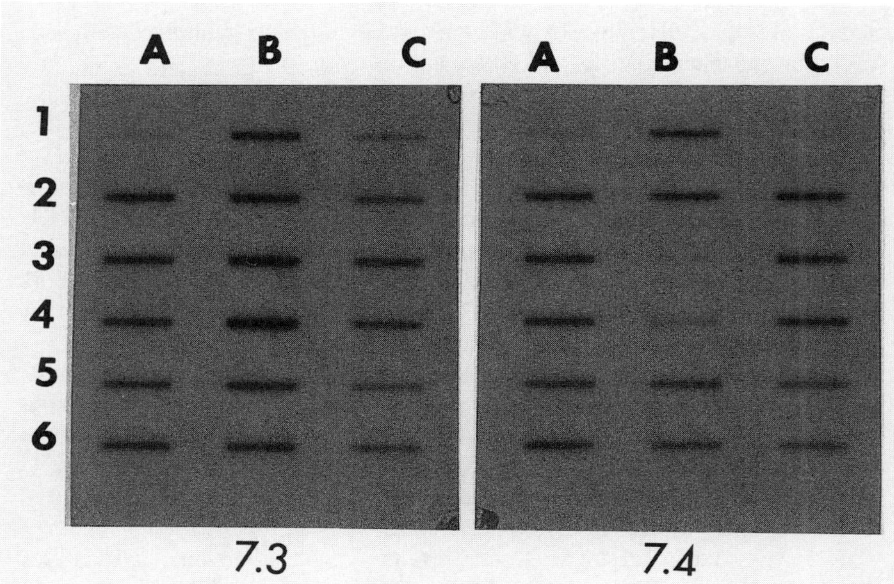

Figure 6 Duplicate slot blots of PCR products amplified with the primers 7.1 and 7.10 for the XbaI RFLP in the factor VIII gene and hybridized with ASO. Hybridization to probe 7.3 corresponds to the presence of the XbaI site and digestion, whereas probe 7.4 hybridizes to sequences lacking this site. **A2–A6** and **C2–C6**. PCR products from the heterozygous fibroblasts. **A1**. Blank. **C1,B3,B4**. Homozygous DNA without restriction site.

Such allele-specific failure of PCR could lead to misdiagnosis of polar bodies and blastomeres in heterozygous conditions. To determine the frequency of allele-specific failure in PCR analysis of single cells, we analyzed 105 single skin fibroblasts heterozygous for the delta-F508 mutation in the CFTR gene, and 64 single skin fibroblasts from an individual heterozygous for the XbaI polymorphic site of the factor VIII gene. Amplification was successful for 78 cells and 43 cells respectively, and, in all cases, both alleles were amplified. The absence of allele-specific PCR failure in 121 consecutive single-cell analyses indicates that diagnostic errors due to allele-specific PCR failure would account for a maximum diagnostic error rate of 0.005 and a minimum error rate of zero.

In all experiments, multiple blank controls were amplified to insure that no contamination of reagents had occurred. Analysis of single cells for the presence of the delta-F508 mutation in the CFTR gene is shown in Figure 5. All heterozygous cells revealed two bands which indicated the successful amplification of both alleles. Figure 6 demonstrates duplicate-slot blots of PCR products amplified by using primers for the Xba1 RFLP in the factor VIII gene which had been hybridized with allele-specific oligonucleotides (ASO) to the plus and the minus alleles. All the PCR products of single cells from a known heterozygous individual hybridized with both ASOs; thus no allele-specific PCR failure has occurred.

Slot Blotting Procedure

Prewet the nylon membrane with distilled water and assemble the blotting apparatus. Denature 5 µl to 30 µl of amplified PCR products in 200 µl of 0.4M NaOH, 25 mM EDTA. Heat the solution for 5 minutes at 95°C and chill on ice. Load each sample twice, rinse the wells with 150 µl of 20 × SSPE and apply vacuum. Take off filter and bake it for 30 minutes at 80°C. Each filter should contain samples from positive and negative controls for each allele.

Prehybridize each filter for at least 30 minutes with 10 ml to 15 ml of prehybridization buffer at 37°C. Add end-label ASO (about 20×10^6 cpm/ml of prehybridization buffer) and hybridize for 2 to 12 hours. Hybridization and wash temperature are indicated in Table IV. Expose filters to X-ray films with intensifying screens at -80°C for 4 to 12 hours. Check with a hand-held GM-counter. If they are still radioactive continue washing till the negatives appear clean.

Table V is a numerical summary of the results of consecutive single-cell analyses of individuals with various genotypes for delta-F508 and the XbaI polymorphism. In the CFTR series, 227 heterozygous cells were analyzed. Amplification was successful for 171 cells (75%). When amplification was successful, the genotype was always correctly identified. The same was true with the analysis of the XbaI mutation for 137 consecutive heterozygous cells, where there was successful amplification of 95 cells (69%).

Table V PCR Analysis of Single Cells of Known Genotype

Delta-F508 mutation in cystic fibrosis transmembrane regulator			
Genotype	CF/CF	CF/N	N/N
Number amplified (%)	51 (81%)	171 (75%)	45 (76%)
CF/CF	51 (100%)	0	0
CF/N	0	171 (100%)	0
N/N	0	0	45 (100%)
Total	63	227	59
Analysis of Xba polymorphic site in factor IX gene			
Genotype	7.4/7.3	7.3	
Number amplified (%)	95 (69%)	43 (67%)	
7.4/7.3	95 (100%)	0	
7.3/7.3	0	43 (100%)	
Total	137	64	

Table VI Multiplex Amplification of Xba Polymorphism and Y-Specific Sequences

Bands visible	Male	Female
Xba + Y (%)	57 (68%)	0
Xba only	0	42 (63%)
Y only	0	0
No bands	27 (32%)	25 (37%)
Total	84	67

In a total of 266 consecutive successful PCR analyses of single cells derived from heterozygous individuals, no instances of allele-specific PCR failure was observed. In cases when both parents are carriers for an autosomal recessive disease, 50% of all embryos would be heterozygous. Therefore, the rate of misdiagnosis following blastomere biopsy for preimplantation genetic analysis due to allele-specific PCR failure is predicted to be less than $1/130 \times 1/2$ or less than 0.0038. For preconception diagnosis using polar body removal and genetic analysis, the rate will be even lower because the fraction of heterozygous polar bodies will vary from a maximum of 50% for telocentric loci to less than 10% for loci located near the centromeric regions. These rates are maximum estimations because we have never actually observed allele-specific PCR failure. The rates are certainly within acceptable limits for a diagnostic test, and will be similar for dominant and X-linked diseases. The introduction of nested primer sets in our analysis of the delta-F508 CFTR mutation has decreased PCR failure rates to less than 5% for the analysis of single cells.

Multiplex PCR of Single Cells

The use of multiplex PCR amplification of repeated sequences specific to the X and Y chromosome has been introduced as an internal control for general PCR failure (Strom et al., 1991). In this study we have compared the efficiency of multiplex PCR

Table VII Multiplex Amplification of X- and Y-Specific Sequences[1]

	Male	Female
X only	0	82 (78%)
Y only	0	0
X and Y	137 (72%)	0
No bands	52 (28%)	23 (22%)
Total	189	105

[1]Some of this data has been published in Strom et al. (1991).

for gender determination using either primers for the Xba1 site in the factor VIII gene, or primers for the X-specific repeated sequences in combination with Y-specific primers. Multiplex PCR using Y-specific and XbaI primers was carried out on 151 single amniocytes obtained by micromanipulation. In addition, 294 cells were subjected to PCR using X-specific and Y-specific multiplex PCR. The results are shown in Tables VI and VII and Figure 7. No diagnostic errors were made in the 445 cells tested. The success rate amplification in XbaI and Y multiplex amplification was 66%, slightly lower than the 74% obtained for the simultaneous X and Y amplification; however, this difference was not statistically significant. Since both methods yielded results with 100% accuracy, we continue to use X- and Y-specific multiplex PCR as the method of choice for gender identification.

Reliability of PCR Analysis in Preimplantation Diagnosis

As mentioned in Chapter 4, this volume, PGD has been carried out in the following genetic disorders: cystic fibrosis (CF) (delta-F508), Tay-Sach's Disease, alpha-1-

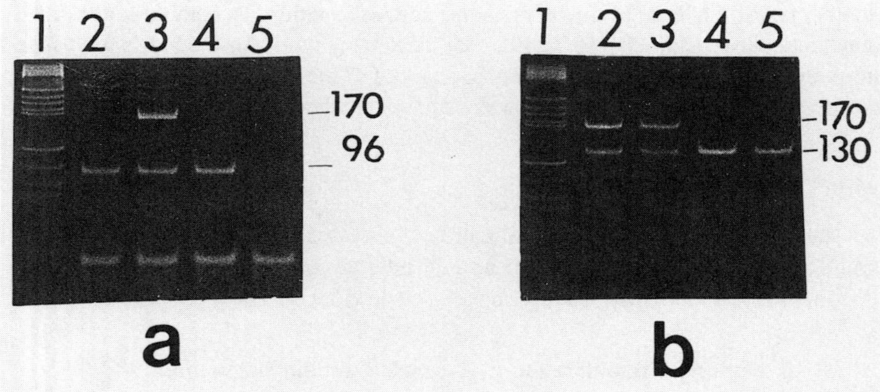

Figure 7 Multiplex PCR of single cells. **a.** Simultaneous amplification of XbaI RFLP site and Y-specific sequence of single amniocytes. 45 cycles of PCR with primers Y1, Y2, and 45 cycles with 7.1, 7.10, as described in Table II. **Lane 1.** Size markers. PBR 322 digested with HaeIII. **Lanes 2 and 4.** Female amniocytes (96 base pair XbaI band). **Lane 3.** Male amniocytes—Y-specific repeats (170 base pairs) and XbaI-specific site (96 base pairs). **Lane 5.** Blank (no DNA added). **b.** Simultaneous amplification of X- and Y-specific sequences of single amniocytes. 45 cycles of PCR were performed with primers X1, X2, and 45 with Y1, Y2; see Table II. **Lane 1.** Size markers. PBR 322 digested with HaeIII. **Lanes 2 and 3.** Male amniocytes—X-specific sequence (130 base pairs), Y-specific sequence (170 base pairs). **Lanes 4 and 5.** Female amniocytes—X-specific repeats (only 130 base pairs).

antitrypsin deficiency, hemophilia, fragile X and Lesch-Nyhan's syndrome. The latter two conditions and one case of hemophilia were approached by gender determination following blastomere biopsy.

In most cases, the preconception genetic analysis by PBR had accurately predicted the genotype of the oocyte, as shown in Tables V to X in Chapter 4, this volume.

However, preconception genetic diagnosis is not possible in a number of situations. In these cases, such as for sex determination in connection with X-linked disorders, blastomere biopsy was performed (Table XI, Chapter 4, this volume). In one case blastomere biopsy and DNA analysis were performed in a couple with CF, where the mother was a carrier of an unknown CF mutation and the father was a carrier of delta-F508. Following embryo biopsy, nine embryos were analyzed; five were found to be homozygous normal and three were found to be heterozygous for delta-F508. The homozygous embryos were transferred and a pregnancy developed. Amniocentesis revealed that the fetus was heterozygous for delta-F508 and linkage analysis demonstrated that the fetus was affected with CF. This couple elected to continue their pregnancy despite the presence of an affected fetus. The child was born without other abnormalities.

There are several possible explanations for this diagnostic error. Allele-specific PCR failure could have occurred, but we feel that this is unlikely given the experiments described above. Contamination with extraneous DNA is another possibility, but this is also unlikely given all the negative controls in the series. Another possibility is that a sperm or maternal coronal cell was inadvertently sampled and the genotype of the sperm, and not the embryo was obtained. This is a definite possibility and has led us to curtail our program of embryo blastomere biopsy for single gene disorder until further data can be obtained. Contamination with sperm would be less of a problem for gender determination. Mistaken inclusion of a extraneous Y-containing sperm would lead to nontransfer of that embryo, but not a misdiagnosis resulting in an affected fetus. Inclusion of an X-containing sperm, may not interfere with the analysis if amplification of the blastomere DNA is proved by reliable method.

At the present time our strategy is to confirm PGD whenever possible. The confirmation of polar body diagnosis was possible either by blastomere biopsy, when embryos were predicted to be affected, or by genotyping the oocytes, if they did not fertilize (Tables VI-VIII, X; Chapter 4, this volume). Confirmation of blastomere diagnosis was also possible when the embryo was found to be affected and was cultured to the blastocyst stage. Finally, the preimplantation diagnosis was confirmed in the products of conception following spontaneous abortion.

The data suggest that preconception genetic diagnosis by polar body removal and PCR analysis can reliably predict the genotype of the oocyte.

References

Coutelle C, Williams C, Handyside A, Hardy K, Winston R, Williamson R (1989): Genetic analysis of DNA from single human oocytes: A model for preimplantation diagnosis of cystic fibrosis. Br Med J 299:22–24.

Dermer SJ, Johnson EM (1988): Rapid DNA analysis of alpha-1-antitrypsin deficiency: Application of an improved method for amplifying mutated gene sequences. Lab Invest 59:403–408.

Faloona F, Weiss S, Ferre F, Mullis K (1990): "PCR" Paper presented at the Sixth International Conference on AIDS, June 20–24, San Francisco, CA.

Handyside AH, Kontogianni EH, Hardy K, Winston RML (1990): Pregnancies from biopsied human preimplantation embryos sexed by Y-specific DNA amplification. Nature 344:768–770.

Handyside AH, Pattinson, JK, Penketh RJA, Delhanty JDA, Winston RML, Tuddenham EGD (1989): Biopsy of human preimplantation embryos and sexing by DNA amplification. Lancet 1:347–349.

Jinno Y, Yoshiura K, Niikawa N (1990): Use of psoralen as extinguisher of contaminated DNA in PCR. Nucleic Acids Res 18:6739.

Kerem B-S, Rommens J, Buchanon JA, Markiewicz D, Cox TK, Chakravarti A, Buchwald M, Tsui L-C (1989): Identification of the cystic fibrosis gene: Genetic analysis. Science 245:1073–1080.

Kogan SC, Doherty M, Gitschier J (1987): An improved method for prenatal diagnosis of genetic diseases by analysis of amplified DNA sequences. New Eng J Med 317:985–990.

Li H, Cui X, Arnheim N (1991): Analysis of DNA sequence variation in single cells. Methods Enzymol 2:49–59.

Li HH, Gyllensten UB, Cui XF, Saikai RK, Ehrlich HA, Arnheim N (1988): Amplification and analysis of DNA sequences in single human sperm and diploid cells. Nature 335:414–417.

Mullis KB, Faloona FA (1987): Specific synthesis of DNA in vitro via a polymerase catalyzed chain reaction. Methods Enzymol 155:335–351.

Myerowitz R, Costigan FC (1988): The major defect in Ashkenazi Jews with Tay-Sach's disease is an insertion in the gene for the alpha-chain of beta-hexosaminidase. J Biol Chem 263:18587–18589.

Navidi W, Arnheim N (1991): Using PCR in preimplantation genetic disease diagnosis. Hum Reprod 6:836–849.

Oleson AE, You L (1989): Use of acylamides for Taq polymerase-dependent amplification of GC-rich target DNA sequences. Abstract, The Fourth San Diego Conference, American Association of Clinical Chemistry.

Perkin Elmer Cetus (Summer 1990): Biotechnology Catalog:p.4.

Pomp D, Medrano JF (1991): Organic solvents as facilitators of polymerase chain reaction. BioTechniques 10:58–59.

Rommens J, Kerem B-S, Greer W, Chang P, Tsui L-C, Ray P (1990): Rapid nonradioactive detection of the major cystic fibrosis mutation. Am J Hum Genet 46,2:395–396.

Sarkar G, Sommer SS (1990a): Shedding light on PCR contamination. Nature 343:27.

Sarkar G, Sommer SS (1991): Parameters affecting susceptibility of PCR contamination to UV inactivation. BioTechniques 10:591–593.

Sarker G, Kapelner S, Sommer SS (1990): Formamide can dramatically improve the specificity of PCR. Nuc Acids Res 18:7465.

Strom CM, Rechitsky S, Verlinsky Y (1991): Reliability of gender determination using the polymerase chain reaction (PCR) for single cells. J In Vitro Fertil Embryo Trans 8:225–229.

Strom CM, Verlinsky Y, Milayeva-Rechitsky S, Evsikov S, Cieslak J, Lifchez A, Valle J, Moise J, Ginsberg N, Applebaum M (1990): Preconception genetic diagnosis for cystic fibrosis by polar body removal and DNA analysis. Lancet 336:306–307.

Triggs-Raine BL, Gravel RA (1990): Diagnostic heteroduplexes: Simple detection of carriers of a 4-bp insertion mutation in Tay-Sach's disease. Am J Hum Genet 46:183–184.

Verlinsky Y, Pergament E, Strom C (1990a): The preimplantation genetic diagnosis of genetic diseases. J In Vitro Fertil and Embryo Trans 7:1–5.

Verlinsky Y, Ginsberg N, Lifchez A, Valle J, Moise J, Strom CM (1990b): Analysis of the first polar body: Preconception genetic diagnosis. Human Reprod 5:826–829.

Waye JS, Willard HF (1985): Chromosome specific alpha satellite DNA: Nucleotide sequence analysis of the 2.0 kilobasepair repeat from the human X chromosome. Nucleic Acids Res 13:2731–2743.

Wolfe J, Darling SM, Erickson RP, Craig DW, Buckle VJ, Rigby PWJ, Willard HF, Goodfellow PN (1985): Isolation and characterization of an alphoid centromeric repeat family from the human Y chromosome. J Mol Biol 182:477–485.

CHAPTER 8

Preimplantation Cytogenetic Analysis

Andrey Dyban, Paul De Sutter, and Yury Verlinsky

Preimplantation cytogenetic analysis may contribute not only to the solving of fundamental theoretical problems in developmental biology and genetics, but can also have diagnostic value for screening and selecting genetically normal oocytes, zygotes or preembryos to be used for clinical purposes. In this chapter we will try to present techniques and summarize data from preimplantation cytogenetic studies in animals and in the human, with special emphasis on their clinical significance and applicability.

Basic Techniques for Chromosomal Preparation From Gametes and Preembryos

In experimental cytogenetic studies carried out in laboratory animals, all stages of spermatogenesis, oogenesis, and early embryonic development can easily be analyzed. Not all stages of gametogenesis and early embryogenesis are available for cytogenetic studies in humans.

Human oogenesis (Fig. 1) starts with the proliferation of primordial germ cells which are located outside the gonad anlage; these cells then migrate to the gonads and undergo several rounds of mitotic division, in which they are transformed to oogonia. In the human, oogonia continue to proliferate until the third month of fetal development. Then a premeiotic round of DNA replication takes place and the oogonia enter meiosis (primary oocytes with a 4c DNA content are formed). From the third to the seventh month of gestation, proliferating oogonia can be found, together with primary oocytes, in the fetal ovary. During this period of development the primary oocytes are at different stages of the first meiotic prophase (leptotene, zygotene, and early pachytene). After the seventh month a first group of oocytes at the late pachytene and early diplotene stage can be observed. Meiosis does not proceed any further and the oocytes are blocked at the late diplotene stage. The oocytes remain at this prophase stage during further fetal development, after birth, and until puberty. In such oocytes a clearly visible nucleus (germinal vesicle) is present. In preovulatory (Graafian) follicles, oocyte maturation starts and meiosis resumes. In these oocytes the germinal vesicle breaks down and the first meiotic division is completed. The chromosome set

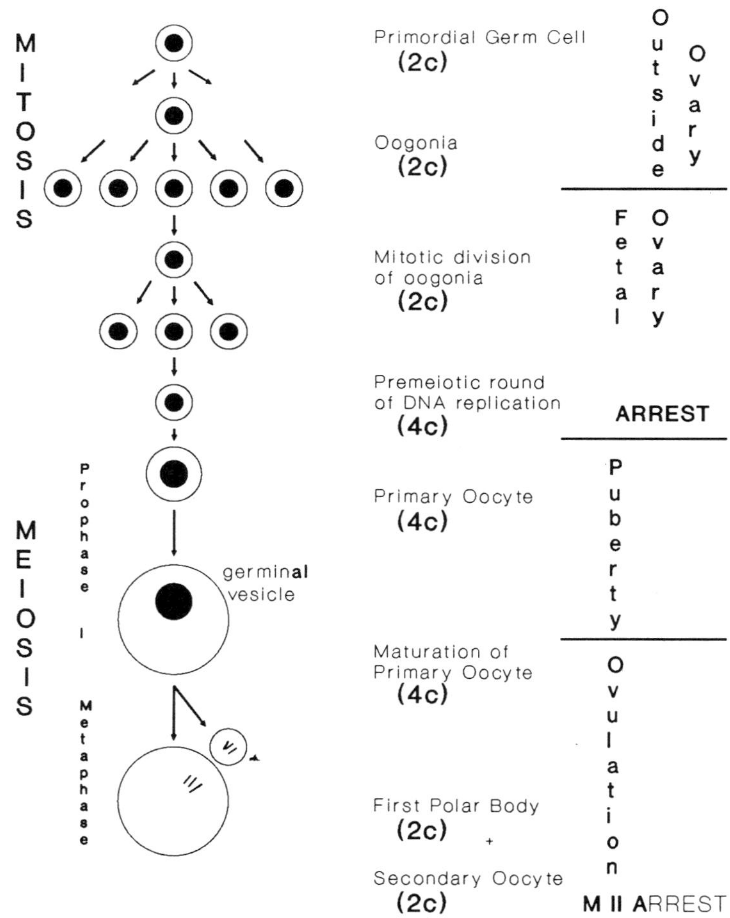

Figure 1 The main stages of mammalian oogenesis. For preimplantation cytogenetic analysis primary maturating oocytes and secondary oocytes can be used.

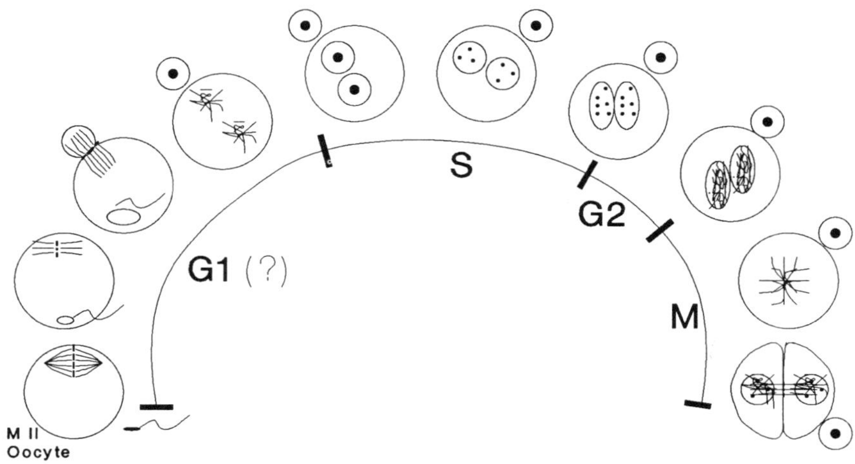

Figure 2 First cell cycle in the fertilized mammalian ovum. During the first cell cycle a real G1-phase does not exist because during this period (from sperm penetration until the appearance of pronuclei) no transcription takes place, but maternal mRNA is translated. Despite the fact that the durations of the S-, G2-, and M-phase are different from those of somatic cells, the processes which take place during these stages are quite analogous.

proceeds from late diplotene via diakinesis to metaphase I. After extrusion of the first polar body, the secondary oocyte is blocked at the second metaphase.

Only after fertilization or artificial activation is the second meiotic division completed; a second polar body is then extruded and the meiotic set of chromosomes will transform into the maternal pronucleus (Fig. 2). After sperm penetration the sperm head decondenses and forms the paternal pronucleus. Both pronuclei enlarge and migrate to the center of the zygote and DNA synthesis takes place. After this round of DNA synthesis, the pronuclei enter into mitosis. The nuclear envelopes disappear and prophase chromosomes become visible in the pronuclei. Then both groups of chromosomes merge in a common diploid metaphase plate. This is followed by anaphase and telophase of the first mitotic division and cleavage of the zygote into two daughter blastomeres (Fig. 2).

It should be stressed that not all stages of human oogenesis can be studied without using material from abortions or ovarian biopsy. For example, potential sources of material for cytogenetic analysis, such as preovulatory oocytes, zygotes and preembryos might be expected from in vitro fertilization (IVF) programs but are not routinely accessible for cytogenetic analysis, since they are used for clinical purposes (fertilization and transfer or cryopreservation) (Table I). Currently polar body removal (PBR) is mainly used for polymerase chain reaction (PCR) analysis and not for cytogenetic analysis. Zygotes and preembryos cultured in vitro can provide very

Table I Material Available for Cytogenetic Analysis Through Human In Vitro Fertilization

Immature oocytes

- germinal vesicle (GV) stage (prophase of the first meiotic division, late diplotene)
- germinal vesicle breakdown (GVBD) (diakinesis)
- metaphase of the first meiotic division (M I)

Mature oocytes

- metaphase of the second meiotic division (M II) + first polar body (PB I)
- isolated PB I (biopsy performed for preimplantation genetic diagnosis)

Oocytes used for insemination in vitro

- remained unfertilized (aged oocytes at M II)
- fertilized oocytes
  - normal zygotes (with male and female pronuclei) + PB II
  - isolated PB II (biopsy performed for preimplantation genetic diagnosis)
  - abnormal fertilization (polyploid zygotes)
  - abortive fertilization: M II chromosomes + prematurely condensed paternal chromosomes, chromatin masses...
- parthenogenetically activated oocytes

Cleaving embryos

- normally developing
- abnormally developing (arrested, fragmented)

Embryonic biopsy

- isolated blastomeres from cleaving embryos
- trophectoderm biopsy from blastocysts

important information, but cytogenetic studies on normally developing human preembryos are currently very difficult to perform due to ethical and other problems. At present, only spare embryos are available from IVF programs, most of them being either triploid, or arrested at the one-cell stage or later. In such material the chromosomes have often started to degenerate and are not suitable for accurate cytogenetic analysis. Notwithstanding all these obstacles, important cytogenetic data can be obtained from IVF material (Table I).

New perspectives in clinical and experimental preimplantation cytogenetic analysis have arisen with the development of micromanipulation techniques. These techniques allow the removal of parts of gametes (polar bodies) or parts of embryos (isolated blastomeres or trophectoderm biopsy) for cytogenetic analysis, without interfering with the developmental potential of gametes or preembryos. In addition to the biopsy technique, isolated blastomeres from animal embryos can be obtained following removal of the zona pellucida by 0.5% pronase or acid Tyrode's solution (pH 2.5). The whole embryo then can be disaggregated into individual cells by mechanical means after incubation in medium free from Ca^{2+} and Mg^{2+} (Ziomek and Johnson, 1980).

Good results can only be expected if the material is fresh or has been kept in optimal culture conditions (temperature, gas mixture, media). Chromosomal preparations from oocytes can be obtained without the use of mitotic arrestants. A sufficiently high yield of metaphase plates from cleaving embryos can only be achieved after a few hours of incubation (at 37°C) in medium containing colcemid or any other mitotic inhibitor, so that most of the blastomeres will be arrested at the metaphase stage. However, we do not recommend the use of a high concentration of colcemid, because this may result in a contraction of the chromosomes which is an obstacle to accurate G-banding. Optimal results can be achieved using a low concentration of colcemid (0.035–0.040 μg/ml).

All currently used methods for obtaining chromosomal preparations from oocytes and preembryos, both in animals and in humans, are based on the method described by Tarkowski (1966), who originally formulated the principles and developed the technique for obtaining chromosomal preparations of preimplantation mouse embryos (Table II). Many modifications of Tarkowski's original method have been described. The gradual fixation technique (Kamiguchi et al., 1976) is believed to produce fewer broken metaphase plates and less artifactual loss of chromosomes (Table III). An advantage of this approach is a more gentle fixation by using several solutions containing different concentrations of methanol and acetic acid. Wramsby and Liedholm (1984) have modified this gradual fixation technique by consecutively using a mixture of distilled water, acetic acid, and ethanol (5:1:4), and acetic acid and

Table II Chromosomal Preparation: Tarkowski's Technique[1]

1. Place the embryo into a hypotonic (1%) sodium citrate solution and leave for 5 to 15 minutes at room temperature. Expanded blastocysts may be kept in the hypotonic solution for up to 15 minutes.
2. Place a microdrop (maximum 0.02 ml) of this solution together with the embryo on a grease-free slide with the help of a mouth-controlled pipette.
3. Expel a few drops (ideally three drops for oocytes) of a mixture of glacial acetic acid and absolute ethyl alcohol (1:3, freshly mixed) from another pipette over the microdrop containing the embryo. The embryo can be observed to flatten and begin to spread. Each consecutive drop should be expelled when the previous one has already spread to such a degree that the embryo again becomes visible on the slide.
4. Air-dry the preparation and examine using a phase contrast microscope and stain.

[1]Tarkowski, 1966.

Table III Chromosomal Preparation: Kamiguchi's[1] Gradual Fixation Technique[2]

1. Put the embryo into hypotonic solution as in Tarkowski's method.
2. Transfer the embryo together with a small amount of hypotonic solution to a mixture of absolute methanol:glacial acetic acid:distilled water (5:1:4).
3. Transfer the embryo after 5 minutes to a grease-free slide and refix by an immediate application of Carnoy's solution.
4. Keep the slide for 20 minutes in a Copplin jar with the same fixative.
5. Dip the slide into a mixture of absolute methanol:glacial acetic acid:distilled water (3:3:1) for 1 minute to help the embryo flatten during the drying process.
6. Air-dry the preparation and examine using a phase contrast microscope and stain.

[1]Kamiguchi et al., 1976
[2]Chandley, 1987

ethanol (1:3), for the fixation of human oocytes. This method limits the risk of breakage of the metaphase plate but leads to poor spreading of the chromosomes, with the result that they are difficult to analyze in detail.

Tarkowski's original technique is very simple but requires considerable skill and experience, without which reliable results are not always easy to obtain. This technique is especially difficult to apply on isolated polar bodies, zona-free embryos, or individual blastomeres. The method described by Dyban (1983, 1991a) is more suitable for such purposes, especially for working with isolated blastomeres or polar bodies (Table IV, Fig. 3). This technique involves first fixing the embryos and then treating them with a softening solution. The structure of the chromosome plates is well preserved and high-quality preparations can routinely be made.

After air-drying the slides are suitable for staining by any method used in modern cytogenetics. For routine purposes, such as counting the number of chromosomes, determining the ploidy, and detecting aneuploidy, Giemsa staining is quite sufficient. Most commercially available Giemsa stock solutions must be freshly diluted in a phosphate buffer (pH 6.8) before use. Excellent results can be obtained by the commercially available modified Giemsa stain (Accustain, Sigma diagnostics # GS-500) diluted 1:50 with deionized water. The slides are stained for 7 minutes in this solution in a Copplin jar at room temperature, then rinsed with running water, and air-dried.

Because mitotic chromosomes from cleaving embryos are less contracted than those in somatic cells, they are suitable for most banding techniques. Very good G-banding can be obtained by the technique described by Evans (1987), or by the much simpler technique routinely used in this institute (Chmura et al., unpublished data, Table V). Until now there have been many technical problems for obtaining reliable G-banding of meiotic chromosomes and this is the reason why accurate karyotyping of second meiotic metaphase oocytes is still a very difficult task. C-banding of meiotic chromosomes is much easier to perform and visualization of the C-band heterochro-

Table IV Chromosomal Preparation: Fixation and Softening Method[1]

1. Hypotonic treatment: Transfer the embryo to a precooled watch glass containing the hypotonic solution, a 1:3 mixture of 1.93% tri-sodium citrate and 0.56% KCl, freshly mixed before use. Both components can be kept in the refrigerator for 10 to 15 days. The duration of the treatment depends on the stage of the embryo. Oocytes are treated for 15 to 20 minutes, isolated blastomeres for 3 to 5 minutes, and morulae for 5 to 10 minutes. Blastocysts should be left in the hypotonic solution for at least 25 minutes or longer (even 1—2 h, but in the refrigerator). All operations are carried out under control of a dissecting microscope, and the embryos are transferred from one solution to another with the help of a mouth-controlled micropipette.
2. Fixation: Place the embryo for 3 to 5 minutes or longer, in a precooled watch glass in a few milliliters of cold fixative (a 1:3 mixture of glacial acetic acid and methanol, kept for at least 1—2 h at -20°C) which dissolves the zona and fixes the embryo. Although the fixative is best prepared on the day of use, it may be kept successfully up to 5 days in the freezer. If the fixative is really cold, the embryos sink to the bottom of the watch glass and do not burst; however, it must not be so cold that the tip of the micropipette freezes before the embryos can be expelled. It is important to carefully observe the embryo during this step since it becomes transparent in the fixative and can be lost.
3. Softening: Transfer the embryo from the fixative to a grease-free slide and add a small drop of softening solution A and observe the outline of the embryo carefully to monitor the degree of spreading. Softening solution A is a fresh 1:1 mixture of methanol, stored in the refrigerator, and 75% acetic acid, stored at room temperature. The optical system of the microscope may need to be adjusted to facilitate observation: a frosted mirror and a clear glass stage are advisable, and the embryos are easier to see if viewed near the boundary between the dark and light parts of the visual field. If the embryo does not spread and flatten, a second drop of softening solution A may be added.
4. Spreading: Add a drop of softening solution B (a fresh 1:1 mixture of methanol and glacial acetic acid) once the embryo is observed to have spread, but before it has dried, in order to achieve final spreading. This can be facilitated by gentle blowing which also hastens drying.
5. Final spreading: Finally, add a drop of fixative (3:1 methanol:glacial acetic acid) to achieve final spreading and drying. Ring the embryo with a glass marker, avoiding the use of a diamond which may pollute the metaphase plates with glass chips. Air-dry quickly by gentle blowing and examine under the phase contrast microscope and stain.

Note: For tiny objects such as isolated blastomeres or polar bodies, better results are obtained when steps 3 and 5 are omitted, and the object is allowed to spread and dry on the slide after application of a small drop of solution B.

[1]Dyban, 1983, 1991a

matin (Chandley, 1987) (Table V) can substantially facilitate the detection of numeric chromosomal aberrations in second meiotic metaphase oocytes.

The dystamycin/4'-6-diamidino-2-phenylindole (DAPI) technique (Schweizer et al., 1978, Table V) provides bright fluorescence at secondary constriction regions of chromosomes 1, 9, and 16, the proximal short arm of chromosome 15, and the distal long arm of the Y-chromosome. This method has successfully been used for the analysis of mitotic chromosomes in cleaving human embryos (Pieters et al., 1992).

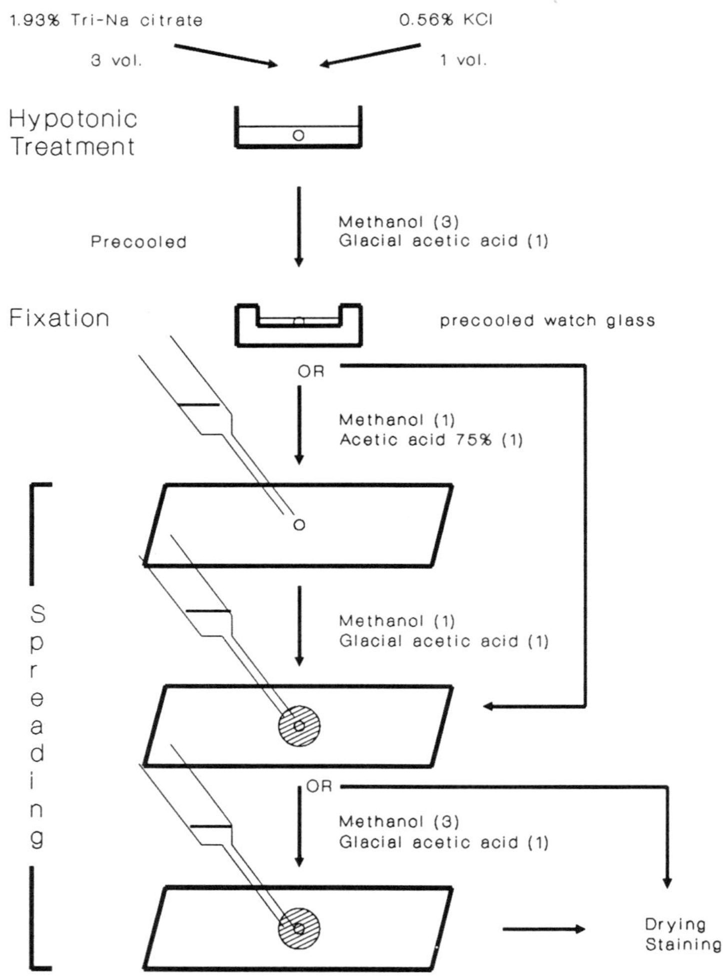

Figure 3 Technique for making chromosomal preparations of gametes and preembryos (Dyban, 1983, 1991a).

Table V Banding Techniques

A. G-banding

1. Age the slides for 7 to 15 days at room temperature, or overnight at 50°C in an incubator.
2. Dip the slides in Hank's balanced salt (HBSS)—pancreatin solution for a few (2–3) seconds; this time is critical and has to be determined empirically, depending on the slide age, embryonic stage, and quality of the metaphase plates. The solution must be freshly prepared by adding 3 ml pancreatin (Gibco 610-5720, keep frozen and thaw immediately prior to use) to 47 ml HBSS, Ca^{2+} and Mg^{2+} free (Gibco 310-4180) at 37°C in a water bath. Adjust the pH with sodium bicarbonate until the color is orange—red orange. This solution can be used for 1 hour, after which it has to be replaced.
2. Rinse quickly in tap water and drain on a paper towel.
3. Stain with Giemsa-Wright for 5 minutes. This stain is freshly prepared by adding 1 ml of prefiltered Giemsa stain (Fisher SO-6-28) and 2 ml of Wright's stock solution [0.8 g Wright's stain (Fisher W-35)] in 480 ml methanol, stirred and ripened for at least 2 days) to 45 ml phosphate buffer (pH 6.8–7.0). The duration of staining is critical and the slide must be checked wet under the microscope until the chromosomes are satisfactorily banded.

B. C-Banding[1] (Chandley, 1987)

1. Keep the slides in 0.2M HCl at room temperature for 1 hour.
2. Rinse with deionized water.
3. Place in 5% barium hydroxide at 50°C for 30 seconds.
4. Rinse with deionized water.
5. Put in 2× standard saline citrate (SSC) (0.3M sodium chloride/0.03M tri-sodium citrate) at 60°C for 1 hour.
6. Rinse with deionized water and stain in Giemsa for 45 minutes.

C. Dystamycin/4'-6-diamidino-2-phenylindole (DAPI) Staining Method[2]

1. Flood the slide with dystamycin A solution (0.1–0.2 mg/ml in McIlvaine's citric acid-Na_2HPO_4 buffer, pH 7.0) and incubate at room temperature in the dark in a wet chamber for 15 minutes. McIlvaine's buffer is prepared by adding 0.63g citric acid and 6.19g sodium phosphate dibasic to 500ml distilled water.
2. Rinse with deionized water.
3. Place a large drop of DAPI solution (0.2–0.4 g/ml in McIlvaine's buffer, pH 7.0) on the slide.
4. Cover the slide and return to the wet chamber in the dark for 30 minutes at room temperature.
5. Rinse with deionized water, mount and seal.

[1]Chandley, 1987.
[2]Schweizer et al., 1978.

Hybridization in situ with radioactive or nonradioactive probes constitutes a promising technique for preimplantation cytogenetic analysis. Chromosome-specific probes are increasingly becoming available and allow for the identification of every individual chromosome. In situ hybridization allows the visualization and location of individual genes in metaphase chromosomes or even interphase nuclei (Lichter et al., 1988). Specific chromosome DNA probes have successfully been used for sexing mouse and human preembryos (Grifo et al., 1991), and human spermatozoa (Pieters et al., 1990; Coonen et al., 1991). Technical details of in situ hybridization are described by Szabo (1989).

Cytogenetic Analysis of the Female Gamete

To date numerous studies have been carried out on unfertilized oocytes from IVF programs. Criteria for failure of fertilization usually include the lack of pronuclear formation and the absence of subsequent cleavage. An appropriate time for fixation of the oocytes is 30 hours after aspiration, since cases of delayed fertilization can then be detected by the delayed appearance of pronuclei after the expulsion of the second polar body. If no pronuclei are detected at that time and only one polar body is present, cleavage will be observed the next day only in rare cases. In most studies, and for practical reasons, however, oocytes are used 48 hours after aspiration, which yields a very high probability of absence of fertilization. Freshly ovulated oocytes are rarely available for cytogenetic analysis, but if oocytes can be analyzed immediately after oocyte aspiration, they must be treated with hyaluronidase (200 IU/ml in culture medium) for a few minutes at 37°C to remove the surrounding cumulus cells. All

Table VI Criteria of Oocyte Maturity[1]

	Mature (Preovulatory)	Immature
Granulosa	Large intercellularspace; cells are loosely connected	Little intercellular space; cells are compact and tightly connected.
Cumulus	Present and expanded	Mostly absent, sometimes present and dense.
Corona	Radiant and expanded	Compact, sometimes absent.
Ooplasm	Round, normal-looking	Darkened by corona cells, round and even, germinal vesicle often visible

[1]Based on Veeck et al., 1983.

oocytes can be treated with 0.5% pronase in culture medium to remove the zona; this is advantageous in case many spermatozoa are attached to the zona.

It is important to collect all possible data available about the history of the oocytes (maturity score at the time of aspiration, the presence of polar bodies) and, of course, relevant patient data such as infertility factors, hormonal treatment, and maternal age. The maturity score is especially important for freshly ovulated oocytes available for analysis, since it directly reflects the nuclear status of the oocyte.

According to Veeck et al. (1983; Veeck, 1986) a mature or preovulatory oocyte (metaphase II) is characterized by: (a) an extruded first polar body; (b) round and even, lightly colored ooplasm, homogeneous in granularity; (c) an expanded and radiant ("sunburst") corona radiata; (d) cumulus cells in a thin expanded matrix; (e) association with follicular granulosa cells which are large, abundant, and present in loosely aggregated sheets (Table VI). The oocyte is considered postmature if the following criteria apply: (a) an intact or fragmented first polar body; (b) ooplasm which may or may not be slightly darkened and/or granular, generally round and even, sometimes with vacuoles; (c) an extremely expanded or clumped darkened corona radiata; (d) a thin and clumping darkened or absent cumulus mass; (e) dark mature granulosa cells.

An intermediate or metaphase I oocyte is characterized by: (a) the absence of a polar body or a germinal vesicle; (b) round and even ooplasm, lightly colored and sometimes slightly granular; (c) a slightly expanded corona radiata; (d) an expanded or dense cumulus mass; (e) mature granulosa cells.

Immature (prophase I) oocytes contain a clearly visible germinal vesicle with a single, refractile nucleolus in their ooplasm, which is sometimes granular and darkened. The corona and cumulus cells, however, may display mature as well as immature characteristics. In the latter case the corona radiata layer usually is very compact, the cumulus mass is not fully expanded, and granulosa cells are small and clumping.

Oocyte Chromosomes

Cytogenetic studies of unfertilized oocytes allow visualization and counting of the number of chromosomes of oocytes arrested at the first or second metaphase. First and second metaphase chromosomes are easily recognizable in human as well as in any other mammalian oocytes. At the first metaphase (Fig. 4A) the chromosome set consists of a haploid number of bivalents (tetrads), the products of pairing of homologous chromosomes. At the second metaphase (Fig. 4C and 4D), the haploid number of chromosomes consists of diads, the products of bivalent disjunction.

If the maternal karyotype is normal the number of bivalents at the first metaphase must be strictly haploid. If, however, at the first metaphase a hypohaploid set is found, or if trivalents, tetravalents and multivalents are present, this indicates that the oocyte is derived from a woman carrying a translocation. This finding can be important for the reproductive prognosis. While hyperhaploidy at the first metaphase can result from the formation of univalents by premature bivalent segregation, it is difficult to exclude the possibilty that univalent formation is due to technical artifacts.

The chromosomes can also be counted and arranged in groups (Denver classification; ISCN, 1985) at the second metaphase (Fig. 5A and 5B), but it is difficult to identify individual chromosomes. It must be mentioned that no more than 50% of all human oocytes are found suitable for cytogenetic analysis (Pellestor, 1991a), since

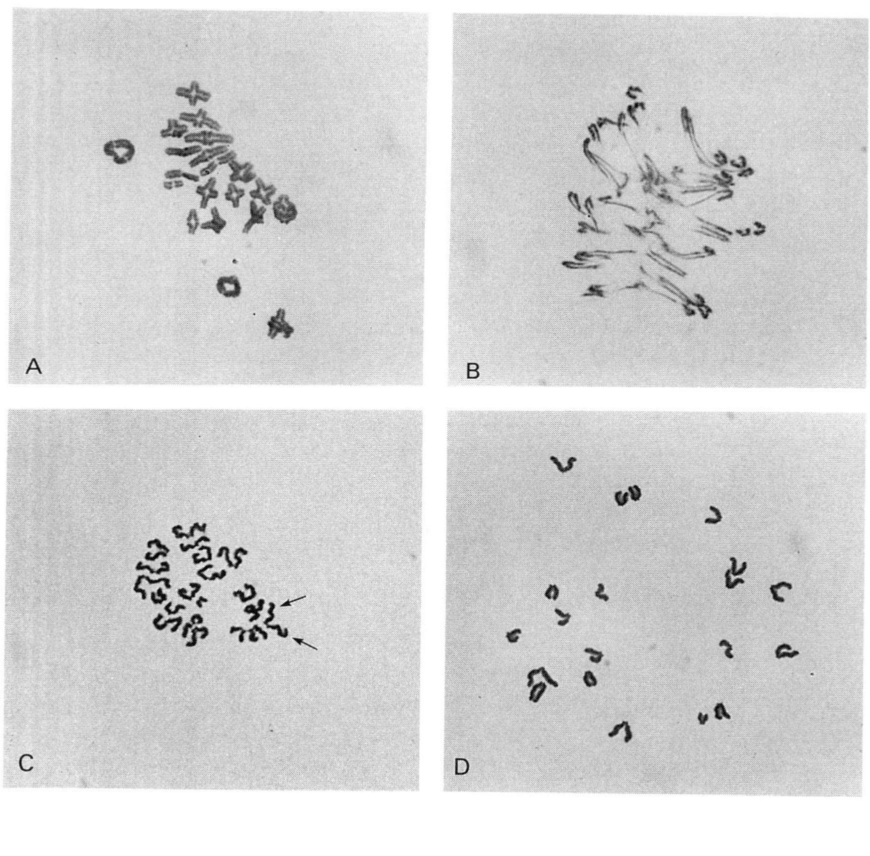

Figure 4 Chromosomes at the first and second meiotic division in mouse oocytes. **A:** First metaphase—twenty bivalents (tetrads) are clearly recognizable. **B:** Anaphase of the first meiotic division—disjunction of bivalents (tetrads) and segregation of homologous chromosomes resulting in two sister haploid groups of chromosomes (diads). **C, D:** Metaphases of the second meiotic division—both plates contain a haploid number (20) of bichromatid chromosomes. Early second metaphase (C): each chromosome consists of two coiled chromatids (arrows). Late second metaphase (D): the chromatids are less coiled.

many oocytes show broken metaphase plates, and the absence or overlapping of chromosomes. Some of these oocytes can only be scored as being grossly haploid or polyploid. It seems that supression of first polar body extrusion occurs at a high rate in human oogenesis, at least after hormonal stimulation. For instance, a diploid number of chromosomes at the second metaphase was found in 6% of oocytes, in a cytogenetic study of 764 unfertilized oocytes (De Sutter, 1991). Fertilization of such oocytes, that is with a nonreduced number of chromosomes, will lead to digynic triploidy, with the formation of one paternal and two maternal pronuclei.

Aneuploidy rates vary in most literature reports, possibly due to differences in the techniques used and in errors occurring at fixation (scattering of chromosomes) or in the analysis of the slides due to overlapping of chromosomes (De Sutter et al., 1991a). The approach most often used to calculate the aneuploidy rate in human oocytes consists of doubling the incidence of hyperhaploid oocytes, while excluding the hypohaploid ones, which may reflect artificial loss of chromosomes. A more precise way to estimate the nondisjunction at the first meiotic division would be to determine the number of chromosomes, not only in the oocyte, but also in the corresponding first polar body (see below). This approach has not yet been used in experimental and clinical cytogenetics.

Initial studies reported aneuploidy rates varying from 8% (Van Blerkom and

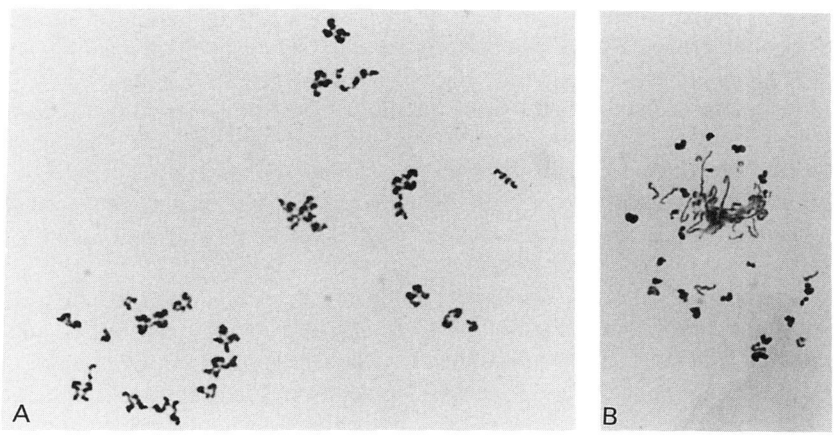

Figure 5 Chromosomes at the second meiotic metaphase in human oocytes. **A:** Presumably hyperhaploid chromosome complement (n > 23). Because, in some chromosomes, premature chromatid separation has occurred, it is difficult to evaluate exactly the real number of bichromatid chromosomes. **B:** A maternal group of meiotic chromosomes (highly contracted) is merged in a common metaphase plate with a group of less contracted and weakly stained paternally derived prematurely condensed chromosomes (PCC).

Henry, 1988) to 47% (Wramsby and Fredga, 1987). De Sutter (1991) found an aneuploidy rate of 23.4%, which is close to the average aneuploidy rate of 22.8% in unfertilized human oocytes as reported by Pellestor, (1991a); the rate of structural anomalies in this review was 1.2%. It has to be mentioned that excluding the hypohaploid oocytes in calculating the rate of aneuploidy ignores the occurrence of anaphase lagging (Martin, 1984), which probably is considerable in human oocytes at the first and second meiotic division. In fact, Van Blerkom and Henry (1988) have observed that even in freshly ovulated oocytes some chromosomes can be found detached from the metaphase spindle scattered in the cytoplasm. These chromosomes are likely to be lost at the completion of the second meiotic division, leading to aneuploidy in the zygote. Nondisjunction at the second meiotic division and anaphase lag will therefore lead to a higher aneuploidy rate than would be calculated from the analysis of unfertilized oocytes arrested at the second metaphase.

The First Polar Body

In most mammals including humans, the first polar body contains chromosomes which do not form a real metaphase plate, and does not contain a spindle. The chromosomes are usually scattered in the cytoplasm from the beginning of the formation until degeneration of the first polar body occurs. In most strains of mice, the first polar body usually survives for only a few hours and disappears during, or soon after, the second meiotic division. There are some data supporting the assumption that the first polar body can survive longer and can even divide, but this has been observed only in some strains of mice (for review see Kaufman, 1983).

The changes in the first polar body of human oocytes have not been described and it is not known how long it survives and when exactly the degeneration process starts either in vivo or in vitro. From our observations (unpublished data) it seems that the human first polar body is more stable than that of the mouse, and that it can persist not only through the second meiotic division but also for many hours after fertilization.

As mentioned above, the counting of the number of chromosomes in the first polar body would improve the estimation of nondisjunction in human and other mammalian oocytes. So far all cytogenetic studies have been performed only by counting the second metaphase oocyte chromosomes. In this laboratory the cytogenetic technique has been improved and adjusted to obtain high quality metaphase plates from the first polar body, in the mouse as well as in humans.

We have observed that the first polar body appears firmly attached to the oocyte immediately after extrusion, and that the spindle with midbodies can be visualized at that time. The chromosomes are uncountable and tightly connected to each other at this stage, which resembles a telophase. After 2 to 3 hours of in vitro culture, individual chromosomes of the first polar body are recognizable. If the polar body is analyzed at this stage, the chromosomes can be counted exactly in the same way as second metaphase oocyte chromosomes. This stage lasts for 2 to 3 hours, and during this period it is possible to see that all chromosomes of the first polar body consist of two chromatids. Later (6–7 h after extrusion), the degeneration of the polar body starts, and the chromosomes gradually lose their individuality to merge into a common chromatin mass. So, the period during which cytogenetic analysis of the first polar body is possible in the mouse is rather short (from 3 to 5 h after extrusion). We have found that it is much easier to obtain good chromosomal preparations from the first polar body in mouse oocytes cultured in vitro, than in oocytes in which the polar body had been extruded in vivo and which were recovered from the oviduct after ovulation.

Figure 6A shows an example of a mouse oocyte containing a hypohaploid chromosome complement (n = 19) and the corresponding first polar body with a hyperhaploid number of chromosomes (n = 21). Since both sets together form a diploid complement (n = 40), this is an obvious example of nondisjunction that was only discovered because the polar body chromosomes were analyzed together with the oocyte.

In the human the first polar body is more resistant and it persists for a much longer period of time than in the mouse. If the chromosomal structural changes follow the same progression as in the mouse, there may be a certain lapse of time during which accurate cytogenetic analysis of the human first polar body is possible. We have tried

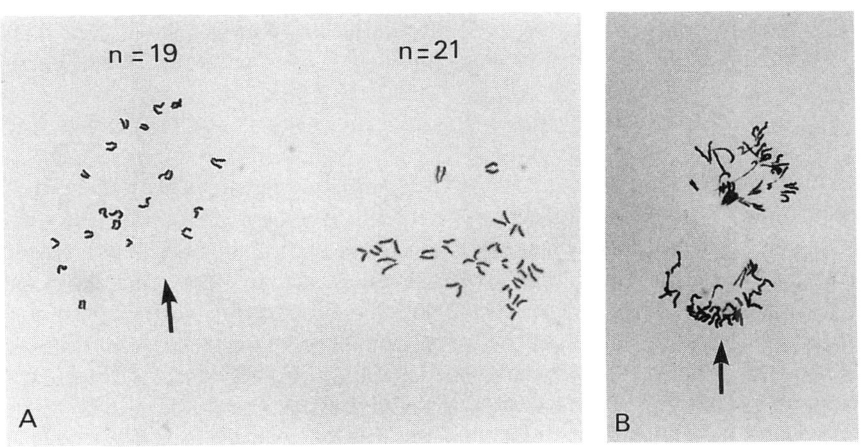

Figure 6 Chromosome sets from the first polar body and the corresponding oocyte. **A:** Malsegregation of one chromosome at the first meiotic division in the mouse. The oocyte (arrow) contains a hypohaploid set (n = 19) of chromosomes, whereas the complementary first polar body contains a hyperhaploid number of chromosomes (n = 21). **B:** Chromosome complements of a human oocyte (arrow) and its first polar body.

to obtain metaphase chromosome preparations from human first polar bodies using IVF oocytes 24 hours after aspiration and were able to get a metaphase chromosome set with a countable number of chromosomes in the first polar body (Fig. 6B).

After 48 hours of in vitro culture, however, the first polar body chromosomes have usually degenerated. If it is possible to find chromosomes of the first polar body at this stage, they resemble second metaphase chromosomes, but are more poorly defined, having a fuzzy outline. They are often found arranged in a circular fashion. Their C-heterochromatin region is sometimes stained more deeply than in oocyte chromosomes (Fig. 7). In most oocytes, however, only remnants of the polar body are found and accurate analysis is impossible.

Our observations suggest that the human first polar body is, in principle, suitable for cytogenetic analysis. At the same time we feel that the existing micromanipulation techniques for first polar body removal must be adjusted so that the chromosomes will be better preserved. More studies are needed to determine the best period of time for the first polar body chromosomes to be analyzed. Although this approach needs further elaborate research, cytogenetic analysis of the first polar body can be very important, not only for a more accurate evaluation of the rate of meiotic nondisjunction, but also in preimplantation genetic diagnosis (PGD). It has been shown that 80% of D and G trisomies are of maternal origin and that 80% of these result from first meiotic nondisjunction (Hassold and Matsuyama, 1979). Using DNA polymorphisms, Antonarakis et al. (1992) have found that 77.1% of maternal trisomy 21 originates from malsegregation at meiosis I, whereas 22.9% is the result of second meiotic nondisjunction. This is why cytogenetic analysis of the first polar body might be valuable for screening patients at risk for the production of aneuploid gametes due to maternal age or to a previous history of trisomy or recurrent abortion.

The Second Polar Body

The second polar body is extruded when the oocyte has been activated by the penetration of sperm (fertilization) or by artificial stimuli (parthenogenetic activation). During the second polar body extrusion, its chromosome set progresses from the anaphase and telophase of the second meiotic division to an interphase, and a visible nucleus is formed. The second polar body can survive much longer than the first polar body. In mice it can be observed until the 2- to 4-cell stage or even later. During the whole period of its survival, the second polar body remains arrested at the interphase state. Although DNA synthesis can take place, the second polar body never enters into mitosis (for review see Kaufman, 1983; Dyban and Baranov, 1978). This is why direct analysis of the second polar body is only possible using interphase cytogenetics, PCR, and molecular biological techniques.

At the same time, the visualization of the second polar body chromosome set can substantially contribute to the study of nondisjunction, not only at the first, but also at the second meiotic division, i.e., at fertilization. According to Modlinski and

McLaren (1980), this idea was formulated by C. Ford. for testing this idea in mouse experiments, Modlinski and McLaren (1980) successfully transferred the second polar body nucleus into a zygote, which under the influence of the zygote cytoplasm transformed into a pronucleus, synthesized DNA and entered the first mitotic division. Despite the fact that the quality of the chromosomal preparation did not allow karyotyping, this work proved that second polar body metaphase chromosomes can be obtained and visualized. Moreover, Modlinski and McLaren suggested that chromosomal analysis of the second polar body can be used for selection of human zygotes with a normal karyotype for transfer in IVF programs.

In this laboratory, this approach was successfully modified, using electrofusion instead of nuclear transplantation (Evsikov et al., unpublished). Mouse second polar bodies were fused, not only with intact, but also with enucleated zygotes, as well as with zygotes from which the maternal pronucleus was removed. In most cases the second polar body nucleus proceeded to the first mitotic metaphase; in some cases the product of the fusion developed until the blastocyst stage. High-quality metaphase chromosome plates derived from the second polar body were obtained. Most of these plates were quite suitable for detailed cytogenetic analysis. These data show that this approach can be used for cytogenetic analysis of the human second polar body.

Recently, a more simple and reliable technique for the visualization of the

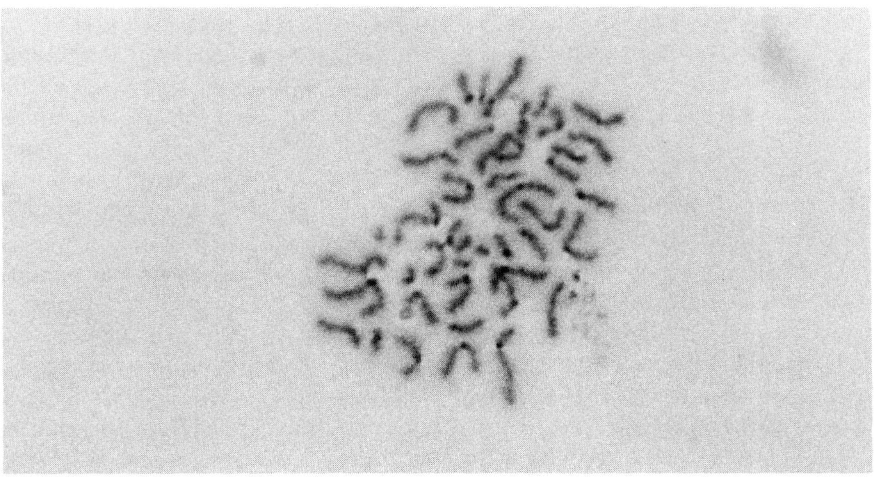

Figure 7 Chromosome set from an isolated human first polar body. Some chromosomes are bichromatid; in others, chromatid separation has taken place. In most chromosomes centromeric heterochromatin is recognizable as dark dots.

chromosomes of the second polar body has been developed. After treatment of one-cell stage mouse embryos with okadaic acid (a specific inhibitor of phosphates 1 and 2A), premature chromosome condensation was obtained, not only in the pronuclei but also in the nucleus of the second polar body. These chromosomes were typically unichromatid G1 prematurely condensed chromosomes (G1-PCC). Using the fixation and softening method it was possible to obtain high-quality preparations which were suitable, not only for counting the number of chromosomes, but also for recognizing structural chromosomal abnormalities, especially after C- and G-banding (Dyban et al., 1992). The efficiency of this technique seems to be very high if the timing of the treatment by okadaic acid is correct.

Removal and analysis of both the first and the second polar body can enhance the sensitivity of the genetic screening and optimize selection of normal embryos in women at risk, as not only nondisjunction at the first but also at the second meiotic division can be detected.

Chromosomal Anomalies in Human Gametes and Factors Influencing Aneuploidy Rates

Much data has been accumulated on the occurrence of chromosome anomalies in human spermatozoa since Yanagimachi and coworkers (Yanagimachi et al., 1976; Rudak et al., 1978; Yanagimachi, 1984) proposed the use of interspecific fertilization of zona-free hamster oocytes by human spermatozoa. Before the introduction of this new method, information could only be obtained through testicular biopsy.

From studies performed by Martin (1990) on more than 5,000 sperm chromosome complements, it was found that 9.4% of human spermatozoa showed structural abnormalities and 4.2% were aneuploid. An excess of hypohaploid over hyperhaploid complements was found. The conservative estimate of aneuploidy (by doubling the frequency of hyperhaploidy) was calculated to be 1.4%, which is much lower than the aneuploidy rates found in human oocytes. Analysis of the frequency of aneuploidy for different chromosomes in spermatozoa showed that chromosomes 1 and 21, and the sex chromosomes, were more predisposed to nondisjunction than the other chromosomes, since more hyperhaploidy was found for these chromosomes (Martin, 1991). Pellestor (1991b) reviewed the main cytogenetic studies carried out on human oocytes and spermatozoa, and found that, in human spermatozoa, group A chromosomes were less prone to nondisjunction than expected, and that all other groups showed an equal distribution of nondisjunction, as expected if nondisjunction were a random event. His results are not in conformity with the original findings of Martin (1991) on this point, but it must be said that Pellestor (1991b) pooled several studies which may have been performed in different ways, and and in which individual chromosomes may not always have been identified.

In oocytes Pellestor found that the frequency of hypohaploidy was not statistically different from the frequency of hyperhaploidy. In oocytes aneuploidy is more frequently observed than structural abnormalities, and attempts have been made to determine which chromosomes are most often involved in this process. Although individual chromosomes cannot be reliably identified by the present techniques, it seems that the acrocentric chromosomes from the D and G groups have a predisposition for nondisjunction (Pellestor, 1991a), a fact which suggests that nondisjunction is not a random event in female meiosis.

There have been several studies on the effect of various clinical factors on the aneuploidy rates in human oocytes. However, in a multicenter study analyzing 316 oocytes, only maternal age has been identified as a factor which significantly influences aneuploidy rates in human oocytes (Plachot et al., 1988). This correlates well with epidemiological data regarding chromosomal anomalies in spontaneous abortions (Boué and Boué, 1973; Hassold et al., 1980). Other studies, however, have not detected any significant differences in oocyte aneuploidy rates as a function of maternal age (Pellestor and Sèle, 1988; Djalali et al., 1988).

The influence of the type of hormonal stimulation used to induce superovulation has not been proven to be important, either in the study by Plachot et al., or in a study comparing two types of gonadotropin-releasing hormone (GnRH) analogs (Tejada et al., 1991). On the other hand, using a specially designed mathematical model (De Sutter et al., 1991a) to minimize the influence of artifacts and errors, De Sutter et al. (1992a) have shown that hormonal stimulation after pituitary suppression by goserelin yields a higher rate of aneuploidy in human oocytes than stimulation by clomiphene citrate (CC) combined with human menopausal gonadotropin (hMG). Other studies have shown that CC-hMG stimulation leads to a larger number of immature oocytes than GnRH agonists, without differences in aneuploidy rates (Pieters et al., 1991). However, it must be kept in mind that different criteria are used to decide on the optimal timing of oocyte aspiration in different stimulation schemes, so that comparison of oocyte maturity scores may not be appropriate. Tarin and Pellicer (1990) found more diploid oocytes in women from whom a large number of oocytes was obtained after GnRH agonist stimulation than in women without GnRH agonist treatment. and they concluded that the occurrence of more immature oocytes could explain the lower fertilization and implantation rates found in these "very good responders" (Pellicer et al., 1989). De Sutter (1991) also noted that pregnancy rates drop if more than 15 oocytes are obtained after GNRH agonist stimulation. In this study, the finding of a higher aneuploidy rate after using GnRH agonists seems to confirm the hypothesis, postulated by Wramsby et al. (1987), that ovarian stimulation, leading to an increased number of oocytes, could be responsible for the maturation of chromosomally abnormal gametes which normally would have undergone atresia.

Very few data on oocytes from unstimulated cycles are available, but some studies have shown a very low aneuploidy rate in these oocytes (Van Blerkom, 1991), a result which indicates that hormonal stimulation probably is responsible for a large number of the observed aneuploid IVF oocytes.

The question remains whether the results regarding unfertilized oocytes can be extrapolated to the overall population of oocytes. If the answer to this question is positive, the chromosome complement of the oocyte would not seem to interfere with its fertilization process. If, on the other hand, as has been proven for oocyte maturity, the unfertilized oocytes are abnormal to a larger extent than fertilized oocytes, this abnormality must somewhere be correlated to the failure of fertilization. An answer to this question cannot be found in the literature, since the conclusions from different studies are in conflict. A few cytogenetic studies have shown similar aneuploidy rates in freshly ovulated oocytes and in unfertilized oocytes (Wramsby et al., 1987; Van Blerkom and Henry, 1988), but they are based on a rather small number of preovulatory oocytes. These findings would suggest that unfertilized oocytes indeed reflect the total oocyte pool of a patient and that there is no correlation between oocyte aneuploidy and fertilizability. On the other hand, there are some indications that the type of infertility problem of a couple influences the rate of aneuploidy in unfertilized oocytes. Zenzes et al. (1992) have observed that some patients have many more aneuploid oocytes than others, so that oocyte chromosome anomalies seem to be strongly patient related. In couples with a male infertility factor, lower aneuploidy rates among unfertilized oocytes are found than in couples where the infertility problem is a tubal factor (Pellestor and Sèle, 1988). Since fertilization rates are known to be higher in the absence of a male factor, it can be expected that oocytes which remained unfertilized are to some extent responsible for the failure of their own fertilization. The finding of higher aneuploidy rates in these oocytes supports the hypothesis that the chromosome complement of the oocyte influences its fertilizability (Pellestor and Sèle, 1988; De Sutter et al., 1991b), since there is no reason to believe that all oocytes in tubal factor patients would show higher aneuploidy rates than those in male factor patients. More studies are definitely needed to elucidate this point.

Cytogenetic Analysis of Human Zygotes and Preembryos

Cytogenetic Observations Related to Fertilization

In most mammals including man, the fertilization process has been studied in detail and divided into definite stages (for review see Yanagimachi, 1984; Wassarman, 1987). Fertilization starts when a sperm penetrates the ovum (gamete fusion or syngamy), and ends when a common metaphase plate is formed (parental genome merging or karyogamy), and the ovum starts to divide (Fig. 8A and B). During the first cell cycle three basic processes can be distinguished: first, meiosis of the ovum is completed, i.e., the M II chromosomes are separated and half are extruded in the

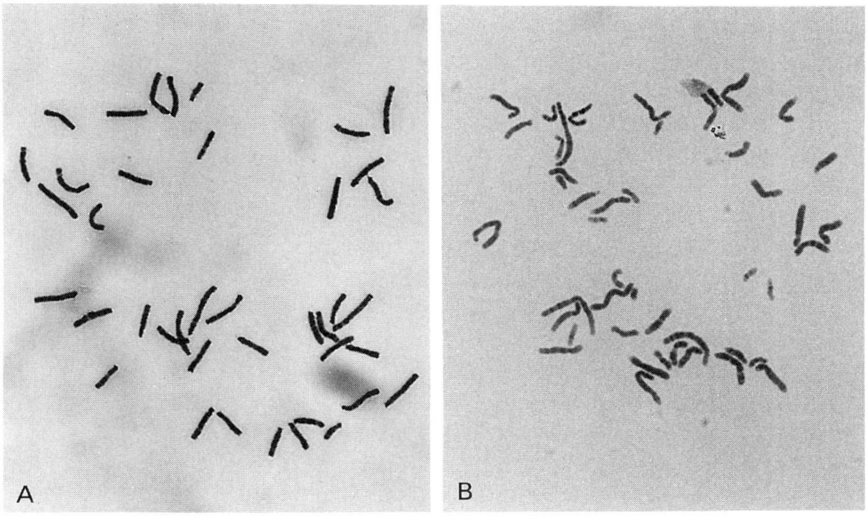

Figure 8 Metaphases of the first cleavage division. **A:** Mouse zygote. The paternal and maternal sets of chromosomes are merged into a common diploid (2n = 40) metaphase plate. **B:** Human zygote. Diploid metaphase (2n = 46) resulting from the mixing of the paternal and maternal chromosome sets.

second polar body; second, maternal and paternal pronuclei are formed; and third, the chromosomes of the pronuclei unite in a common diploid metaphase plate, and the ovum divides into two blastomeres (Fig. 2).

The transformations of the maternal chromosome complement and the sperm head into pronuclei have been investigated in detail and this process is the same in all mammals including man. It must be stressed that the chronology of this process is very well known in mice and other laboratory animals but has been poorly studied in humans. Therefore the duration of the phases of the first cell cycle (G1, S, G2, and M) is unknown in the human, especially since it seems that some zygotes can enter the first mitotic division earlier (24 h after insemination) and some much later (up to 48 h after insemination) than average (30 h after insemination).

It must be noted that, in the mouse, the paternal pronucleus starts to become visible before the maternal pronucleus, and that both may differ in size. In human zygotes a clear difference in size between both pronuclei can also be observed; this difference may reflect the asynchrony in the formation and development of the paternal and maternal pronucleus. DNA replication takes place in each pronucleus independently and, after the S-phase, the DNA content has doubled (changed from 1c to 2c) in both pronuclei, which originally were haploid. The prophase and prometaphase transitions of the pronuclei take place without mixing the chromosomes originating from the sperm and the oocyte (Donahue, 1972; Kaufman, 1973), so that the parental sets line up as segregated haploid groups, which will only later form a common diploid metaphase plate. The formation of this common metaphase plate is essential for the normal segregation of chromosomes during the first cleavage division.

There are differences in chromosomal spiralization between the maternal and paternal chromosome sets. This heterocyclicity was first noted during the early embryogenesis of insects and fish (Prokofeva-Belgovskaya, 1981), and has also been observed in mouse zygotes, where the maternal set of chromosomes is more spiralized than the paternal one (Donahue, 1972; Kaufman, 1973; Dyban and Baranov, 1987). Our observations support the idea that the same chromosomal heterocyclicity can be seen in human zygotes.

It seems logical to assume that the heterocyclicity of the parental sets of chromosomes in the zygote is determined by the initial state of the parental and maternal genetic material. At the time of fertilization the paternal set forms condensed chromatin in the sperm head, whereas the maternal genome consists of second metaphase meiotic chromosomes and needs more time to complete meiosis before pronucleus formation can start. At the same time, there are some data (Dyban, 1987) which indicate that there is a regionalization in the ooplasm of factors which determine the rate of chromosomal transformation, so that different concentrations of these unknown factors result in different rates of pronuclear development. This hypothesis of an uneven distribution of such ooplasmic factors has been supported by the study of parthenogenetic diploid one-cell stage mouse embryos. Despite the fact that both pronuclei were of maternal origin in these embryos, the chromosomal transformation was asynchronous and one chromosome set was more spiralized than the other (Dyban and Noniashvili, 1985; Dyban, 1987, 1988). We have observed the same picture in artificially activated human parthenogenetic embryos (De Sutter et al., 1992b) (Fig. 9).

As all different stages of pronucleus formation and different stages of the first mitotic division (from prophase to metaphase, anaphase, and telophase) may be expected in the cytogenetic analysis of human zygotes it is important to take into consideration the exact developmental age of the zygote. For example, the finding of two distinct interphase nuclei or two haploid groups of prometaphase chromosomes can be interpreted as normal—depending on the developmental age, i.e., stage of fertilization—or, on the contrary, as a sign of developmental arrest or even abortive fertilization.

In some in vitro inseminated oocytes, fertilization takes place incompletely. In such oocytes, not only the maternal set of meiotic chromosomes, but also some structures which are derived from the sperm head can be found. Single chromatin masses and different stages of early pronuclear degeneration belonging to the paternal components of abortive fertilization can be observed, even without the presence of maternal meiotic chromosomes. Probably in these cases the maternal set has been extruded.

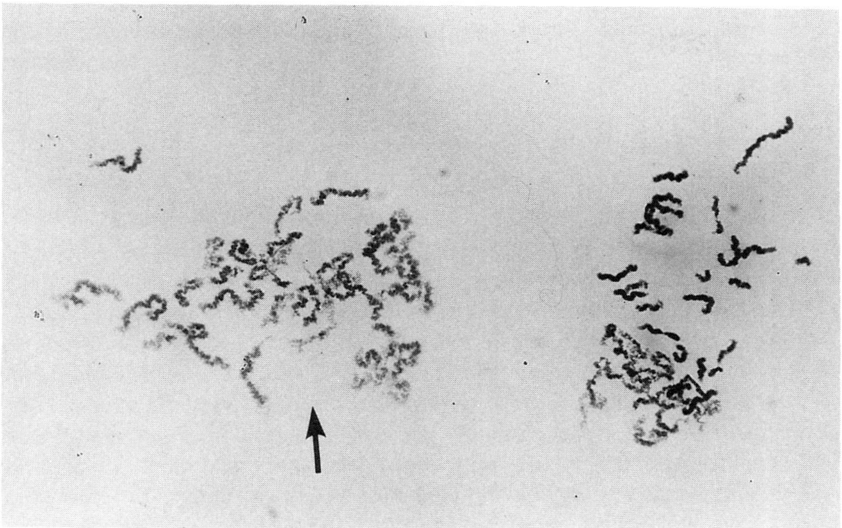

Figure 9 Late prophase or early prometaphase in a human parthenogenetically activated oocyte. One group consists of coiled, slightly condensed chromosomes (arrow) whereas in the other group heterochromatization of chromosomes is clearly visible.

One of the typical signs of abortive fertilization is the presence of a group of prematurely condensed chromosomes (PCC) which have been described long ago (Brachet, 1922) and are a well-known phenomenon in fusion experiments of interphase cells with mitotic cells (Johnson and Rao, 1970). PCC are found in 7% (De Sutter, 1991) to 30% (Pieters et al., 1989) of supposedly unfertilized oocytes. Depending on the stage of the interphase nucleus which condenses prematurely (G1-,S-, or G2-phase), the PCC will have different morphologies. In some unfertilized human oocytes (Schmiady and Kentenich, 1989), PCC are typical elongated unichromatid chromosomes (G1-PCC, Figs. 5B and 10), and the identification of the Y-chromosome by G-banding has confirmed the paternal origin of these chromosomes (Schmiady et al, 1986). They are thought to be the result of sperm having penetrated a cytoplasmic immature oocyte in which some chromosome condensing factors had not disappeared. Although sperm penetration takes place in this kind of oocyte, the oocytes fail to be activated and remain arrested at the second metaphase. PCC seem to occur more frequently in first metaphase (34%) than in second metaphase oocytes (14%) (Plachot, 1991). This finding has been confirmed by the peculiar response of these PCC-containing oocytes to activation agents such as puromycin (De Sutter et al., 1992b). Clumps of scattered chromatin were found in 2% of 764 unfertilized oocytes analyzed (De Sutter, 1991). Some oocytes containing meiotic oocyte chromosomes or PCC are also found to contain chromatin masses. The exact origin of these chromatin masses is not known, but they might be due to abortive fertilization of the oocytes.

Chromosomal Constitution of One-Cell Stage and Cleaving Embryos

Normal zygotes contain one maternal and one paternal pronucleus and have full developmental potential. In clinical IVF programs such zygotes are usually further cultured and used for transfer or cryopreservation. Cytogenetic aspects of cleavage and development of such human embryos have been reported (Plachot et al., 1987, 1989; Wimmers and Van der Merwe, 1988; Papadopoulos et al., 1989). From animal data it is well known that at the early stages of development, many mammalian embryos are chromosomally abnormal (for review see Dyban and Baranov, 1987). Bearing in mind the high aneuploidy rates in human oogenesis and spermatogenesis and the probability of mitotic nondisjunction during cleavage, the rate of aneuploidy in early human embryos may be expected to be very high. In fact, 16% to 40% of cleaving human embryos that resulted from phenotypically normal zygotes showed chromosome anomalies (Plachot et al., 1987, 1989; Papadopoulos et al., 1989). Diploid/haploid and triploid/haploid mosaicism is one of the major anomalies

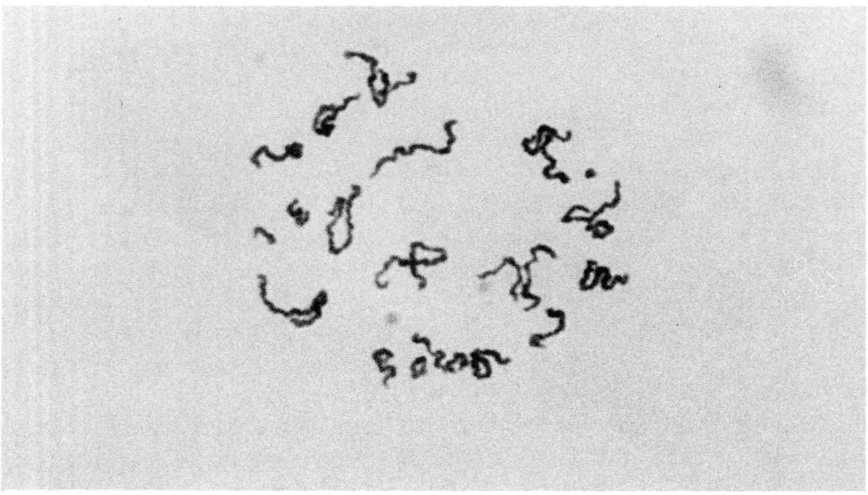

Figure 10 Paternal set of 23 prematurely condensed chromosomes (PCC), found in a presumably unfertilized human oocyte.

encountered. Such changes in the karyotype can result from DNA replication errors, nuclear extrusion and/or failure of cytokinesis during cleavage.

Because it has been shown that in the mouse any trisomy is compatible with preimplantation development, it may also be the case in humans (Dyban and Baranov, 1987; Dyban, 1991b). Monosomy of most chromosomes is also compatible with preimplantation development in the mouse, but some monosomies, and all nullisomies, result in early cleavage arrest (for review see Dyban and Baranov, 1987; Dyban, 1991b). In human spontaneous abortions, monosomies are observed more seldom than trisomies and it is suggested that all monosomic human embryos are dying at the early stages of development, probably at or soon after implantation.

Originally Plachot et al. (1987) could not detect a significant correlation between the cytogenetic constitution and the morphology of cleaving human embryos, but this observation was made on a rather limited number of embryos. Moreover, most studies were performed on embryos which have been rejected from transfer or cryopreservation because of their morphological appearance. However, Ma et al. (1990) have observed a significantly higher rate of chromosomal anomalies in embryos with an abnormal morphology. It thus remains unclear whether the expression of chromosomal anomalies in cleaving human embryos differs from that in animal embryos.

Haploidy. Since there are no facts in favor of the assumption that a male pronucleus can be formed without the formation of the female pronucleus, single-pronucleate oocytes are believed to be the result of parthenogenetic activation. This activation can occur spontaneously or be induced by a wide variety of agents, such as improper handling or temperature fluctuations. Single-pronucleate oocytes can also be the result of extrusion of the maternal set of chromosomes from a zygote and the formation of a single paternal pronucleus. Cases of diploid human androgenesis are found in later stages of gestation (Szulman and Surti, 1978, 1984), but androgenetic haploid human embryos have never been described (Dyban and Baranov, 1987).

Plachot et al. (1988, 1989) have calculated the frequency of single-pronucleate oocytes to be 1.6% after in vitro insemination. It is, however, still unclear whether these oocytes are really parthenogenetic, gynogenetic (i.e., activated by sperm, without the participation of the sperm in the pronuclear formation), or androgenetic embryos. Plachot (1991) studied the further development of such oocytes and found that 20% were able to reach the blastocyst stage. More than 50% of the embryos resulting from single-pronucleate oocytes were in fact found to be diploid, indicating that some of these single-pronucleate oocytes formed a diploid nucleus, or that diploidization has taken place at a later stage. In parthenogenetically activated haploid mouse embryos, diploid metaphases have been observed at later stages of cleavage, indicating that these embryos have diploidized (Tarkowski, 1977; Kaufman, 1983; Dyban and Noniashvili, 1985). These facts indicate that in mammalian

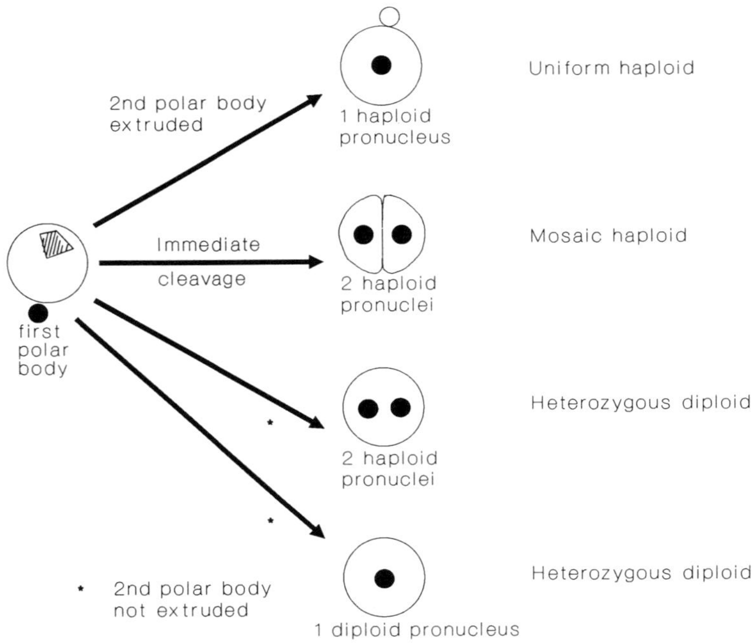

Figure 11 Main routes of parthenogenetic development in the mouse. Two types of haploid and two types of diploid parthenogenetic embryos can be obtained by artificial activation with various agents.

embryos a haploid karyotype is unstable, and this is why all attempts to obtain haploid cell lines from mouse parthenogenetic embryos have failed (Graham, 1977).

Analysis of haploid metaphases in mouse parthenogenones has shown that these chromosomes are predisposed to structural aberration. Isochromosomes, dicentrics, microchromosomes with centric fragments, and chromatid breaks are not uncommon findings in parthenogenones, compared to diploid embryos (Dyban and Baranov, 1987; Dyban, 1988, 1991b).

In the mouse the different routes of parthenogenetic development (Fig. 11) have been studied in detail (Graham, 1974; Tarkowski, 1975; Whittingham, 1980; Kaufman, 1983; Dyban and Baranov, 1987): immediate cleavage into two haploid cells (mosaic haploids), formation of a haploid single-pronucleate embryo with extrusion of the second polar body (uniform haploids), formation of a diploid single-pronucleate embryo with retention of the second polar body (one class of heterozygous diploids) and, finally, the formation of a diploid bi-pronucleate embryo with retention of the second polar body (another class of heterozygous diploids). From the results of activation experiments in human oocytes by Ca-ionophore A23187 (Winston et al., 1991) and puromycin (De Sutter et al., 1992b), it seems that all four routes occur in the human as well, so that the estimated frequency of 1.6% is probably an underestimate for this phenomenon. The parthenogenone with two pronuclei, in particular, has to be distinguished from the product of regular fertilization in IVF programs. Parthenogenesis, gynogenesis, and androgenesis in the human are poorly understood to date, and more studies are required to evaluate their contribution to failure of early embryonic development.

Artificial parthenogenetic activation of human oocytes provides a valuable model for the study of early embryonic development and may in the future be useful for cytogenetic analysis of unfertilized human oocytes. Parthenogenetic activation of unfertilized human oocytes leads to the formation of mitotic metaphase plates which can be analyzed by most cytogenetic techniques used for mitotic cells (Fig. 12A and B).

Triploidy. Triploidy is one of the most frequent spontaneous genome aberrations in embryos of different mammalian species, including the human. Triploidy may result from dispermic fertilization (diandry) or fertilization of a nonreduced ovum (digyny). Because triploid embryos can be obtained quite easily in mouse experiments, their preimplantation and postimplantation development has been studied in detail. It has been shown that in this species a triploid zygote (diandric as well as digynic) can cleave normally, form a blastocyst, implant, and develop until early

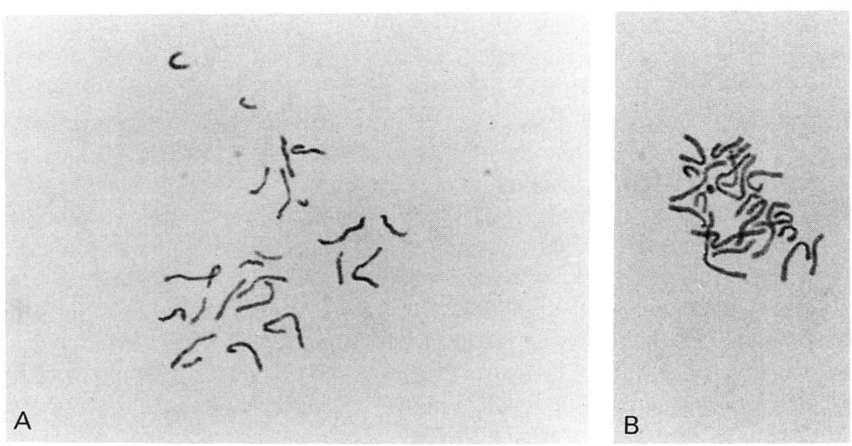

Figure 12 Haploid mitotic metaphase plates in parthenogenetically activated human oocytes. Both plates are suitable for banding and karyotyping. **A:** Well-spread haploid (n=23) metaphase plate. **B:** Hypohaploid (n = 21) set of mitotic chromosomes.

organogenesis. During all these stages the triploid karyotype is preserved and no cases of diploidization have been reported (for review see Dyban and Baranov, 1987).

Triploidy is found in about 4% to 6% of all human IVF zygotes (Tejada et al., 1991, Plachot et al., 1989). Polyspermic fertilization (diandry) is more frequently found in immature oocytes (Rudak et al., 1984). The cortical granule reaction which normally forms a block against polyspermy is abnormal in immature oocytes, since the cortical granules have not yet reached the subcortical zone of the ooplasm (Trounson et al., 1982). A high sperm concentration in the insemination medium has also been held responsible for polyspermic fertilization (Edwards, 1982). Another mechanism for diandry is fertilization of an oocyte by a diploid sperm cell. In the human, there is a natural selection in vivo against diploid sperm cells, which are eliminated during the sperm migration to the ampulla of the oviduct, due to their abnormal motility. During sperm preparation for IVF, this selection is probably bypassed, and this explains why the incidence of fertilization by diploid sperm cells is higher in vitro than in vivo (Santalo et al., 1986).

Another source of triploid zygotes are oocytes that contain a diploid set of maternal chromosomes and are fertilized by one sperm (digyny). A diploid set of maternal chromosomes derives from the failure of the second meiotic division as a result of the suppression of second polar body extrusion. Digynic triploid zygotes can easily be obtained in the mouse, using cytochalasin B or D which depolymerizes the microfilaments and suppresses cytokinesis (Balakier and Tarkowski, 1976; Niemierko and Opas, 1978).

The importance of oocyte factors for the occurrence of triploidy is illustrated by the findings of Maudlin and Fraser (1977), who reported a simple dose-response relationship between the incidence of triploidy and hormonal stimulation (dose of pregnant mare's serum gonadotropin) and of Wentz et al. (1983), who reported a higher rate of polyspermy in human IVF after using HMG for hormonal stimulation than after using the combination of CC and HMG. De Sutter (1991) showed a higher frequency of triploidy after using GNRH agonists than after CC and HMG. The same difference in triploidy rates was observed by Plachot et al. (1988), who compared HMG alone to the combination of GNRH agonists and HMG. These findings, however, may be explained by a direct correlation between a high fertilization rate and a high incidence of triploidy. Correspondingly, a lower rate of triploidy has been found in couples with male infertility and thus lower fertilization rates. Cytogenetic analysis of zygotes with three real pronuclei has revealed that all of them are indeed triploid (Rudak et al., 1984). In some cases, however, vacuoles can be mistaken for pronuclei and the number of pronuclei can be miscalculated. Cytogenetic analysis of such zygotes will therefore reveal diploidy.

The developmental potential of human triploid zygotes is much lower than of diploid zygotes. Eighteen percent of triploids do not cleave in vitro, in contrast to 4% of diploid zygotes (Plachot et al., 1989). In arrested tri-pronuclear zygotes, all kinds of cytogenetic pictures can be observed. Sometimes an asynchronous breakdown of the different nuclear membranes takes place, and after fixation both condensed chromosomes and chromatin masses can be observed. De Sutter (1991; De Sutter et al., 1991a) observed an abnormal number of chromosomes in analyzable metaphase plates in this kind of zygote more frequently than in unfertilized oocytes. In contrast to embryos from triploid mouse zygotes (see above), the majority of embryos resulting from human triploid zygotes are found to be diploid or diploid/triploid mosaics (71%, Pieters et al., 1992). There are indications that such changes in the karyotype are the result of tripolar mitosis. Triploid zygotes can follow different routes of development: tripolar mitosis leading to a mosaic diploid embryo; bipolar mitosis giving rise to a uniform triploid embryo; extrusion of one of the pronuclei leading to a diploid embryo. Depending on whether the triploid is digynic or diandric, and on which pronucleus is extruded, a perfectly normal diploid embryo, or an androgenetic or gynogenetic diploid embryo will be formed (Plachot, 1991; Pieters, 1992). Tripolar mitosis, however, has not yet been described in cleaving mouse embryos. In the mouse and other animals, triploid zygotes almost always cleave to two cells, but in the human the cleavage of genuine triploid zygotes into three cells can be observed quite often (Kola et al., 1987). In this laboratory, we have repeatedly observed three pronuclei in live triploid zygotes using an inverted microscope. In addition, we have confirmed that some such zygotes can cleave not only into two but also into three cells. Cytogenetic analysis revealed a diploid karyotype in these blastomeres.

Sathananthan et al. (1991) have recently shown that a human sperm contributes centrioles to the oocyte at fertilization. Paternal centrioles then may participate in the organization of the spindle and determine the pattern of cleavage. This is quite different from the case in mouse zygotes, in which paternal centrioles do not participate in the organization of the mitotic spindle (Szöllösi et al., 1972). If the observation of Sathananthan et al. is confirmed, a different cleavage pattern between digynic and diandric triploids can be expected: only dispermic triploids can directly cleave into three cells, whereas digynic triploids may follow the normal cleavage patterns. Future research will show if such criteria can be used for differentiating between diandric and digynic human triploids at the beginning of their development.

A Possibility for Diagnostic Preimplantation Cytogenetic Analysis

Experiments in the mouse and other mammals (rabbit, sheep, cow) have shown with certainty that blastomeres of cleaving embryos are pluripotent and that removal of one or even more cells from the morula does not interfere with subsequent developmental potential (for review see Papaioannou and Ebert, 1986). Live offspring have been obtained after blastomere removal in many species. This approach is now routinely applied in animal breeding (for review see First, 1991) and provides the scientific basis for using isolated blastomeres for cytogenetic analysis.

The first successful attempt to karyotype microsurgically isolated blastomeres for detecting monosomy and trisomy was performed long ago in mouse embryos (Severova and Dyban, 1984). Karyotype abnormalities (trisomy and/or monosomy for chromosome 15 and 17) were detected in blastomeres removed from embryos at the 4-cell stage. The three remaining blastomeres were cultured in vitro up to the blastocyst stage and used for chromosomal preparation. In this way the influence of an aneuploid karyotype on the rate of cleavage and blastocyst formation was accurately studied. The potential implications of such an approach for preimplantation cytogenetic diagnosis seem to be obvious (Bacchus and Buselmaier, 1988; Roberts et al., 1990), as the determination of karyotype peculiarities of live human embryos will make it possible to select for transfer only embryos without chromosomal abnormalities. Some of the current limitations of these approaches are purely technical. First, obtaining chromosomal preparations from single embryonic cells is still rather difficult and not only must high-quality equipment and reagents be available but also considerable technical skill is needed for these operations. The interpretation of the results can also be difficult because of the occurance of chromosomal mosaicism in human embryonic development. To detect chromosomal mosaicism, more than one metaphase per embryo must be available. However, individual blastomeres at the morula stage do not have synchronized cell cycles, and removal of two or more blastomeres may not always help in diagnosing mosaicism. Therefore, biopsy and analysis at the blastocyst stage may be a solution since more cells can be obtained; however, further studies are needed to test these approaches for cytogenetic analysis in preimplantation human development.

For IVF, accurate preimplantation cytogenetic diagnosis will make it possible to prevent fertilization and pregnancy failure that is determined by chromosomal abnormalities, and to avoid the transfer of cytogenetically affected embryos. However, many problems still remain to be solved and many efforts are needed before preimplantation cytogenetic analysis will be routinely used for diagnostic purposes.

References

Antonarakis SE, Petersen MB, McInnis MG, Adelsberger PA, Schinzel AA, Binkert F, Pangalos C, Raoul O, Slaugenhaupt SA, Hafez M, Cohen MM, Roulson D, Schwartz S, Mikkelsen M, Tranebjaerg L, Greenberg F, Hoar DI, Rudd NL, Warren AC, Metaxotou C, Bartsocas C, Chakravarti A (1992): The meiotic stage of nondisjunction in trisomy 21: Determination by using DNA polymorphisms. Am J Hum Genet 50:544–550.

Bacchus C, Buselmaier W (1988): Blastomere karyotyping and transfer of chromosomally selected embryos. Hum Genet 80:333–336.

Balakier H, Tarkowski AK (1976): Diploid parthenogenetic mouse embryos produced by heat-shock and cytochalasin B. J Embryol Exp Morphol 35:25–39.

Boué JG, Boué A (1973): Increased frequency of chromosomal anomalies in abortions after induced ovulation. Lancet 7804:679–680.

Brachet A (1922): Recherches sur la fécondation prématurée de l'oeuf d'oursin. Arch Biol 32:205–244.

Chandley AC (1987): Meiotic analysis in germ cells of man and the mouse. In Monk M (ed): "Mammalian Development: A Practical Approach." Oxford: IRL Press, pp. 71–91.

Coonen E, Pieters MH, Dumoulin JC, Meyer H, Evers JL, Ramaekers FC, Geraedts JP (1991): Nonisotopic in situ hybridization as a method for nondisjunction studies in human spermatozoa. Mol Reprod Dev 28:18–22.

De Sutter P (1991): Investigation of determining factors for in vitro fertilization of human oocytes. Cytogenetic analysis. Postdoctoral Thesis. Ghent, Belgium: University of Ghent, pp. 72-130.

De Sutter P, Dhont M, Verschraegen-Spae MR, Steyaert H, Corijn W, Leroy J, Vandekerckhove D (1991a): Chromosome analysis of human oocytes failing to fertilize in vitro: A mathematical model for the estimation of the first meiotic non-disjunction frequency. Hum Reprod 6:550-554.

De Sutter P, Dhont M, Vanluchene E, Vandekerckhove D (1991b): Correlations between follicular fluid steroid analysis, maturity and cytogenetic analysis of human oocytes which remained unfertilized after in vitro fertilization. Fertil Steril 55:958-963.

De Sutter P, Dhont M, Vandekerckhove D (1992a): Hormonal stimulation for in vitro fertilization: A comparison of fertilization rates and cytogenetic findings in unfertilized oocytes. J Assist Reprod Genet (in press).

De Sutter P, Dozortsev D, Cieslak J, Wolf G, Verlinsky Y, Dyban A (1992b): Parthenogenetic activation of human oocytes by puromycin. J Assist Reprod Genet (in press).

Djalali M, Rosenbusch B, Wolf M, Sterzik K (1988): Cytogenetics of unfertilized human oocytes. J Reprod Fertil 84:647–652.

Donahue RP (1972): Cytogenetic analysis of the first cleavage division in mouse embryos. Proc Nat Acad Sci U S A 69:74–77.

Dyban AP (1983): An improved method for chromosome preparations from preimplantation mammalian embryos, oocytes or isolated blastomeres. Stain Technology 58:69–72.

Dyban AP (1987): Studies of cellular, chromosomal and molecular mechanisms of very early mammalian embryogenesis. Sov Sci Rev F Physiol Gen Biol 1:651–701.

Dyban AP (1988): "Early Mammalian Development." Leningrad: Nauka (in Russian).

Dyban AP (1991a): Reliable technique for chromosomal preparations from mammalian oocytes, preimplantation embryos and isolated blastomeres. In Verlinsky Y, Kuliev A (eds): "Preimplantation Genetics." New York: Plenum Press, pp. 293-298.

Dyban AP (1991b): Experimental cytogenetics of preimplantation development. In Verlinsky Y, Kuliev A (eds): "Preimplantation Genetics." New York:Plenum Press, pp 15-23.

Dyban AP, Baranov VS (1978): Cytogenetics of Mammalian Development. Moscow, Nauka (in Russian).

Dyban AP, Baranov VS (1987): Cytogenetics of Mammalian Embryonic Development. Oxford, Oxford University Press.

Dyban AP, DeSutter P, Dozortsev D, Verlinsky Y (1992): Visualization of the second polar body chromosmoes in fertilized and artificially activated mouse oocytes treated by okadaic acid. J Ass Reprod Genet, in press.

Dyban AP, Noniashvili EM (1985): The factors determining the incidence and the rate of parthenogenetic development in mouse eggs activated by ethyl alcohol treatment. Ontogenez 6:582–597 (in Russian with English summary).

Edwards RG (1982): The case for studying human embryos and their constituent tissues in vitro. In Edwards RG, Purdy JM (eds): "Human Conception in Vitro. Proceedings of the First Bourn Hall Meeting." London: Academic Press, pp. 370–388.

Evans EP (1987): Karyotyping and sexing of gametes, embryos and fetuses and in situ hybridization to chromosomes. In Monk M (ed) "Mammalian Development: A Practical Approach." Oxford: IRL Press, pp. 93–114.

First NL (1991): Manipulation techniques with potential use in animal agriculture. In Verlinsky Y, Kuliev A (eds): "Preimplantation Genetics." New York: Plenum Press, pp. 49–61.

Graham CF (1974): The production of parthenogenetic mammalian embryos and their use in biological research. Biol Rev 49:399-422.

Graham CF (1977): Teratocarcinoma cells and normal mouse embryogenesis. In Sherman SJ (ed): "Concepts in Mammalian Embryogenesis." Cambridge, MA: MIT Press, pp. 315–394.

Grifo JA, Ward DC, Boyle A (1991): In situ hybridization of blastomeres from embryo biopsy. In Verlinsky Y, Kuliev A (eds): "Preimplantation Genetics." New York: Plenum Press, pp. 147–152.

Hassold T, Chen N, Funkhouser J, Joss T, Manuel B, Matsuura J, Matsuyama A, Wilson C, Yamane JA, Jacobs PA (1980): A cytogenetic study of 1000 spontaneous abortions. Ann Hum Genet 44:151–178.

Hassold T, Matsuyama A (1979): Origin of trisomies in human spontaneous abortions. Hum Genet 46:285–294.

ISCN (1985): An international system for human cytogenetic nomenclature: Birth defects. Original Article Series, Vol 21, No 1. New York: The National Foundation.

Johnson RT, Rao PN (1970): Mammalian cell fusion: Induction of premature chromosome condensation in interphase nuclei. Nature 226:717–722.

Kamiguchi Y, Funaki K, Mikamo K (1976): A new technique for chromosome study of murine oocytes. Proc Jap Acad 52:316–321.

Kaufman MH (1973): Timing of the first cleavage division of the mouse and the duration of its component stages: A study of living and fixed eggs. J Cell Sci 13:553–556.

Kaufman MH (1983): "Early Mammalian Development: Parthenogenetic Studies." Cambridge, UK: Cambridge University Press.

Kola I, Trounson AO, Dawson G, Rogers P (1987): Tripronuclear human oocytes: Altered cleavage patterns and subsequent karyotypic analysis of embryos. Biol Reprod 37:395–401.

Lichter PL, Cremer T, Borden J, Manuelidis L, Ward DC (1988): Delineation of individual human chromosomes in metaphase and interphase cells by in situ suppression hybridization using recombinant DNA libraries. Hum Genet 80:224–234.

Ma S, Kalousek DK, Zouves C, Yuen BH, Gomel V, Moon YS (1990): The chromosomal complement of cleaved human embryos resulting from in vitro fertilization. J In Vitro Fertil Embryo Transf 7:16–21.

Martin RH (1984): Comparison of chromosomal abnormalities in hamster egg and human sperm pronuclei. Biol Reprod 31:819–825.

Martin RH (1990): Chromosomal analysis of human spermatozoa. J In Vitro Fertil Embryo Transfer 7:196.

Martin RH (1991): Chromosomal analysis of human spermatozoa. In Verlinsky Y, Kuliev A (eds): "Preimplantation Genetics." New York: Plenum Press, pp. 91–102.

Maudlin I, Fraser L (1977): The effect of PMSG dose on the incidence of chromosomal anomalies in mouse embryos fertilized in vitro. J Reprod Fertil 50:275–280.

Modlinski J, McLaren A (1980): A method for visualizing the chromosomes of the second polar body of the mouse egg. J Embryol Exp Morphol 60:93–97.

Niemierko A, Opas J (1978): Manipulation of ploidy in the mouse. In Daniel JR (ed): "Methods in Mammalian Reproduction." New York: Academic Press, pp. 50–67.

Papadopoulos G, Templeton AA, Risk N, Randall J (1989): The frequency of chromosome anomalies in human preimplantation embryos after in vitro fertilization. Hum Reprod 4:91–98.

Papaioannou VE, Ebert KM (1986): Comparative aspects of embryo manipulation in mammals. In Rossant J, Pedersen R (eds): "Experimental Approaches to Mammalian Embryonic Development." Cambridge, UK: Cambridge University Press, pp. 67–96.

Pellestor F (1991a): Frequency and distribution of aneuploidy in human female gametes. Hum Genet 86:283–288.

Pellestor F (1991b): Differential distribution of aneuploidy in human gametes according to their sex. Hum Reprod 6:1252–1258.

Pellestor F, Sèle B (1988): Assessment of aneuploidy in the human female by using cytogenetics of IVF failures. Am J Hum Genet 42:274–283.

Pellicer A, Ruiz A, Castellvi RM, Catalyud C, Ruiz M, Tarin JJ, Miro F, Bonilla-Musoles F (1989): Is the retrieval of high number of oocytes desirable in patients treated with gonadotrophin-releasing hormone analogues (GnRH-a) and gonadotrophins? Hum Reprod 4:536-540.

Pieters MH, Geraedts JP, Dumoulin JC, Evers JL, Bras M, Kornips FH, Menheere PP (1989): Cytogenetic analysis of in vitro fertilization (IVF) failures. Hum Genet 81:367-370.

Pieters MH, Geraedts JP, Meyer H, Dumoulin JC, Evers JL, Jongbloed RJ, Nederlof PM, van der Flier S (1990): Human gametes and zygotes studied by nonradioactive in situ hybridization. Cytogenet Cell Genet 53:15-19.

Pieters MH, Dumoulin JC, Engelhart CM, Bras M, Evers JL, Geraedts JP (1991): Immaturity and aneuploidy in human oocytes after different stimulation protocols. Fertil Steril 56:306-310.

Pieters MH, Dumoulin JC, Ignoul-Vanvuchelen RC, Bras M, Evers JL, Geraedts JP (1992): Triploidy after in vitro fertilization: Cytogenetic analysis of human zygotes and embryos. J Assist Reprod Genet 9:68–76.

Plachot M, Junca AM, Mandelbaum J, de Grouchy J, Salat-Baroux J, Cohen J (1987): Chromosome investigations in early life. II. Human preimplantation embryos. Hum Reprod 2:29–35.

Plachot M, Veiga A, Montagut J, de Crouchy J, Calderon G, Lepretre S, Junca AM, Santalo J, Carles E, Mandelbaum J, Barri P, Degoy J, Cohen J, Egozcue J, Sabatier JC, Salat-Baroux J (1988): Are clinical and biological IVF parameters correlated with chromosomal disorders in early life: A multicentric study. Hum Reprod 3:627–635.

Plachot M, Mandelbaum J, Junca AM, de Grouchy J, Salat-Baroux J, Cohen J (1989): Cytogenetic analysis and developmental capacity of normal and abnormal embryos after IVF. Hum Reprod 4 (Suppl):99–103.

Plachot M (1991): Chromosome analysis of oocytes and embryos. In Verlinsky Y, Kuliev A (eds): "Preimplantation Genetics." New York: Plenum Press, pp. 103-112.

Prokofeva-Belgovskaya AA (1981): Heterocyclicity of nucleus systems. In Beliaev K (ed) "Genetics and Human Welfare." Moscow: Nauka, pp. 314–318.

Roberts C, Lutjen J, Krzyminska U, O'Neill C (1990): Cytogenetic analysis of biopsied preimplantation mouse embryos: Implications for prenatal diagnosis. Hum Reprod 5:197–202.

Rudak E, Dor J, Mashiach S, Nebel L, Goldman B (1984): Chromosome analysis of multipronuclear human oocytes fertilized in vitro. Fertil Steril 41:528–545.

Rudak E, Jacobs PA, Yanagimachi R (1978): Direct analysis of the chromosome constitution of human spermatozoa. Nature 274:911–913.

Santalo J, Estop AM, Egozcue J (1986): The chromosome complement of first-cleavage mouse embryos after in vitro fertilization. J In Vitro Fert Embryo Transf 3:99–105.

Sathananthan AH, Kola I, Osborne J, Trounson A, Ng SC, Bongso A, Ratnam SS (1991): Centrioles in the beginning of human development. Proc Natl Acad Sci U S A 88:4806–4810.

Schmiady H, Kentenich H (1989): Premature chromosome condensation after in-vitro fertilization. Hum Reprod 4:689-695.

Schmiady H, Sperling K, Kentenich H, Stauber M (1986): Prematurely condensed human sperm chromosomes after in vitro fertilization (IVF). Hum Genet 74:441-443.

Schweizer D, Ambros P, Andrle M (1978): Modification of DAPI banding on human chromosomes by prestaining with a DNA-binding oligopeptide antibiotic, dystamicin A. Exp Cell Res 111:327–332.

Severova EL, Dyban AP (1984): The live selection of early mouse embryos according to sex and karyotype peculiarities. Ontogenez 16:585–591 (in Russian with English summary).

Szabo P (1989): In situ hybridization. In Verma RS, Babu A (eds): "Human Chromosomes. Manual of Basic Techniques." New York: Pergamon Press, pp. 152–165.

Szöllösi D, Calarco P, Donahue R (1972): The spindle pole in early mammalian development. J Cell Sci 11:521–542.

Szulman AE, Surti U (1978): The syndromes of hydatiform mole. I. Cytogenetic and morphologic correlations. Am J Obstet Gynecol 131:665–671.

Szulman AE, Surti U (1984): The syndromes of partial and complete molar gestation. Clin Obstet Gynecol 27:172–180.

Tarin JJ, Pellicer A (1990): Consequences of high ovarian response to gonadotropins: A cytogenetic analysis of unfertilized human oocytes. Fertil Steril 54:665–670.

Tarkowski AK (1966): An air-drying method of chromosome preparations from mouse eggs. Cytogenetics 5:394–400.

Tarkowski AK (1975): Induced parthenogenesis in the mouse. In Markert CL (ed): "33rd Symposium of the Society of Developmental Biology: Developmental Biology of Reproduction." New York: Academic Press, pp. 107-129.

Tarkowski AK (1977): In vitro development of haploid mouse embryos produced by bisection of one-cell fertilized eggs. J Embryol Exp Morphol 38:187–202.

Tejada MI, Mendoza R, Corcostegui B, Benito JA (1991): Chromosome studies in human unfertilized oocytes and uncleaved zygotes after treatment with gonadotropin-releasing hormone analogs. Fertil Steril 56:874–880.

Trounson A, Mohr L, Wood C, Leeton J (1982): Effect of delayed insemination on in vitro fertilization, culture and transfer of human embryos. J Reprod Fertil 64:285–294.

Van Blerkom J (1991): Extrinsic and intrinsic influences on human oocyte and early embryo developmental potential. In Wassarman PM (ed): "Elements of Mammalian Fertilization. Vol 2. Practical Applications." Boca Raton, FL: CRC Press, pp. 81–109.

Van Blerkom J, Henry G (1988): Cytogenetic analysis of living human oocytes: Cellular basis and developmental consequences of perturbations in chromosomal organization and complement. Hum Reprod 3:777–790.

Veeck LL (1986): Atlas of the Human Oocyte and Early Conceptus. Baltimore: Williams and Wilkins.

Veeck LL, Wortham JWE, Witmyer J, Sandow BA, Acosta AA, Garcia JE, Jones GS, Jones HW (1983): Maturation and fertilization of morphologically immature oocytes in a program of in vitro fertilization. Fertil Steril 39:594–602.

Wassarman P (1987): The biology and chemistry of fertilization. Science 235:553–560.

Wentz CA, Repp JE, Maxson WS, Pittaway DE, Torbit CA (1983): The problem of polyspermy in in vitro fertilization. Fertil Steril 40:748–754.

Whittingham DG (1980): Parthenogenesis in mammals. In Finn CA (ed): "Oxford Reviews of Reproductive Biology, Vol 2." Oxford: Oxford University Press, pp. 205-231.

Wimmers MSE, Van der Merwe JV (1988): Chromosome studies on early human embryos fertilized in vitro. Hum Reprod 3:894–900.

Winston N, Johnson M, Pickering S, Braude P (1991): Parthenogenetic activation and development of fresh and aged human oocytes. Fertil Steril 56:904-912.

Wramsby H, Fredga K (1987): Chromosome analysis of human oocytes failing to cleave after insemination in vitro. Hum Reprod 2:137–142.

Wramsby H, Liedholm P (1984): A gradual fixation method for chromosomal preparations of human oocytes. Fertil Steril 41:736–738.

Wramsby H, Fredga K, Liedholm P (1987): Chromosome analysis of human oocytes recovered from preovulatory follicles in stimulated cycles. N Engl J Med 316:121–124.

Yanagimachi R (1984): Zona-free hamster eggs: Their use in assessing fertilizing capacity and examining chromosomes of human spermatozoa. Gamete Res 10:187–232.

Yanagimachi R, Yanagimachi H, Rogers B (1976): The use of zona-free animal ova as a test system for the assessment of the fertilizing capacity of human spermatozoa. Biol Reprod 15:471–476.

Zenzes MT, Wang P, Casper RF (1992): Evidence for maternal predisposition to chromosome aneuploidy in multiple oocytes of some in vitro fertilization patients. Fertil Steril 57:143–149.

Ziomek CA, Johnson MH (1980): Cell surface interaction induces polarization of mouse 8-cell blastomeres at compaction. Cell 21:935–942.

CHAPTER 9

Problems in Preimplantation Genetic Diagnosis and Areas for Future Research

Yury Verlinsky and Anver M. Kuliev

Analysis of present experience shows that preimplantation genetic diagnosis (PGD) is still at the research stage, with many existing problems in the micromanipulation and biopsy of gametes and preembryos, as well as in genetic analysis of the biopsied material. At the moment, DNA analysis by polymerase chain reaction (PCR) is the only acceptable approach for PGD; biochemical methods are not completely reliable, while the possibility of cytogenetic analysis has not yet been demonstrated, except for some preliminary attempts in the application of in situ hybridization techniques in mouse (Grifo et al., 1991) and human preimplantation embryos (Handyside, personal communication).

Preimplantation Diagnosis of Chromosomal Diseases

As described in Chapter 8, this volume, in spite of extensive cytogenetic studies of early embryonic development, including attempts to visualize the chromosomes of the second polar body of the mouse egg (Modlinsky and McLaren, 1980), to karyotype biopsied single mouse and human blastomeres (Severova and Dyban, 1984; Verlinsky et al., 1987; Bacchus and Buselmaier, 1988; Handyside et al., 1989; Kola and Wilton, 1991), and to develop preconception chromosomal analysis based on utilization of the first polar body (Verlinsky et al., 1991), there is still no efficient technique for PGD of chromosomal disorders. At the same time the data available on cytogenetic analysis of unfertilized oocytes and preimplantation embryos from IVF programs, which are summarized in Chapter 8, this volume, demonstrate the importance of developing preconception and preembryo diagnosis of chromosomal disorders. It is obvious that the frequency of chromosomal abnormalities in preimplantation development is very high (about 28%), making cytogenetic analysis of great value in any IVF program, as chromosomal abnormalities may be one of the most important causes of the low success rate of IVF. Fetal loss due to chromosomal abnormalities from the time of fertilization to the time of birth, according to this data, is as follows: The theoretical rate of chromosomal abnormalities at fertilization is about 40%, taking into account both the rate of aneuploidies in oocytes and sperm, and fertilization related abnormalities. As can be expected from the mouse data (Gropp, 1975; Epstein, 1985; Dyban and Baranov, 1987), most of these abnormalities will be compatible with cleavage. At the same time, a strong selection against chromosomal abnormalities is obvious during implantation, as almost half of aneuploid preimplantation embryos are lost. A further loss of chromosomal abnormalities after implantation is realized in spontaneous abortions, over half of which are known to be due to chromosomal abnormalities. As a result of this selection against chromosomal abnormalities, both before and after implantation, only 0.6% of newborns have chromosomal diseases, and most of these lead to serious disabilities that are incompatible even with early childhood.

Analysis of cytogenetic data in oocytes, sperm, and early preimplantation embryos (Chapter 8, this volume) also suggests the relevance of preimplantation chromosomal studies, not only for couples at high risk of conceiving a child with chromosomal disorders, such as couples carrying balanced translocations, but also for couples with any other indication for preimplantation genetic analysis. It seems reasonable to suggest that cytogenetic investigation would also be very useful in IVF programs, to prevent the transfer of chromosomally abnormal embryos that would lead to embryonic loss via spontaneous abortions.

Identification of morphological markers for cytogenetically defective early human embryos will make it possible to exclude chromosomally abnormal embryos from transfer. One of the recent publications in this area has demonstrated that about 30% of fragmented human embryos appeared to be chromosomally abnormal (Bongso et al., 1991). This is in agreement with earlier reported data, which revealed chromosomal abnormalities in 19% of fragmented embryos, compared to 11% of healthy ones (Plachot et al., 1987). It is of interest that only grade 2 embryos implant and yield pregnancies in IVF programs, and that only a certain proportion of fragmented embryos are able to implant when kept in vitro for 4 to 5 days. Only about 10% of fragmented embryos are able to cleave regularly, to cavitate, and to form blastocysts with inner cell masses (Bongso et al., 1991). Thus, a poor outcome for implantation of fragmented embryos may be due to chromosomal abnormalities.

However, before cytogenetic methods can be implemented for PGD, many technical and theoretical problems have to be resolved. Much research is still needed to achieve high resolution cytogenetic analysis of polar bodies. Although cytogenetic analysis of single human blastomeres seems realistic, the success rate is still too low to implement such analysis in practice. In addition, cytogenetic analysis of embryos after IVF raises the important problem of chromosomal mosaicism, which is as high as 7% (Plachot et al., 1989). In such cases the karyotype of a single blastomere or of a trophectoderm cell might not reflect the karyotype of the embryo. A high proportion of mosaicism (about 20%) was found in fragmented embryos (Bongso et al., 1991) and may lead to a different outcome of the pregnancy depending on whether the inner cell mass or the trophectoderm will be formed from chromosomally abnormal blastomeres. It is possible that embryos in which the embryo proper is derived from abnormal blastomeres either fail to implant or eliminate very early, while embryos in which abnormal blastomeres form trophectoderm, present further problems of interpretation in chorionic villus sampling (CVS) for prenatal diagnosis. Therefore, in prenatal diagnosis at the first and second trimester of pregnancy by CVS, mosaicism will present a source of potential misinterpretation, raising questions on the diagnostic accuracy in preimplantation cytogenetic diagnosis.

Another approach to preimplantation diagnosis of chromosomal abnormalities will be the use of in situ hybridization or the study of DNA polymorphisms by locus-specific probes or chromosomal painting, which make it possible to also utilize the interphase cells. With progress in identifying chromosome-specific probes and with highly polymorphic sites for each chromosome, it might be realistic to screen gametes and biopsied cells of preembryos for aneuploidies and structural chromosomal abnormalities. However, the data available show that in situ hybridization using chromosome- and gene-specific probes do not reveal a signal in every cell, with only about 80% to 90% of cells showing detectable hybridization. Therefore, PGD based on in situ hybridization of a single cell might not be reliable, and might be a realistic possibility only with trophectoderm cells biopsied from blastocysts. Moreover, even with blastocyst biopsy it would be difficult to exclude a chromosomal mosaicism, which, as mentioned previously, is not particularly rare in preimplantation development. Consequently, before in situ hybridization can be reliably used for PGD of chromosomal disorders, more research will be needed to improve the accuracy of this powerful technology.

Preimplantation Enzyme Analysis

Inherited enzyme defects cause severe chronic disease leading, in most of the cases, to death in early childhood. Since, in many of these genetic disorders, the recurrence risk is as high as 25%, preimplantation enzyme analysis might be an important option for those couples who cannot accept prenatal diagnosis and the subsequent elective abortion of an affected pregnancy.

Preimplantation genetic diagnosis of the enzyme defect for Lesch-Nyhan's syndrome (deficiency of hypoxanthine phosphoribosyl transferase, HPRT) was first demonstrated in a mouse model by trophectoderm biopsy (Monk et al., 1988). However, human embryonic genome activation was suggested to occur no earlier than at the 8-cell stage, compared to mouse embryonic genome activation occurring as early as at the 2-cell stage (Braude et al., 1979, 1988; Flach et al., 1982; Tesarik et al., 1988). Braude et al. (1989) measured HPRT activity in 46 preimplantation human embryos cultured in vitro up to the blastocyst stage, but, as no significant rise was found, measurement of HPRT cannot be used for diagnostic purposes. The average levels of HPRT activity for 4-cell, morula, and blastocyst stages were similar to those found in unfertilized eggs; thus either the measurable enzyme activity was maternal in origin, or any new activity could not be revealed because it was masked by partial breakdown in maternally derived enzyme which is not easily distinguishable from embryonic enzyme. The authors also found a substantial variation in enzyme activity between individual embryos, and blastomeres taken from the same embryo, a fact which leaves open the question of what are appropriate normal enzyme levels corresponding preimplantation stage of development (Brande,1991). Similar variations were found in the data obtained by Sermon et al. (1992) on the use of microassay of hexosaminidase for PGD of Tay-Sach's disease.

Further research on the feasibility of using single cells of preimplantation embryos for diagnosing enzyme deficiencies will show if new technology needs to be developed to realize the PGD of human enzyme defects.

Accuracy of Preimplantation DNA Analysis

DNA analysis for preconception and preimplantation diagnosis has become realistic with the application of PCR, which makes it possible to amplify minute quantities of DNA obtained from a single cell (Li et al., 1988; Coutelle et al., 1989; Handyside et al., 1989; Monk and Holding, 1990; Strom et al., 1990). However, this increases the chance of DNA contamination, which is the most difficult problem in PGD at the moment (see Chapter 7, this volume). Statistical analysis based on the amplification of 708 single-sperm samples showed that every sample has about a 5% probability of DNA contamination (Cui et al., 1989). As the usual techniques for preventing DNA contamination are ineffective when analyzing single cells, specially designed decontamination procedures have to be applied which are based on the elimination of double-stranded DNA sequences (Porter-Jordan and Canarett, 1990; Bianchi et al., 1990; Strom et al., 1990). In addition, possible sources of contamination have to be carefully excluded from the embryology reagents, water, salt solutions, oligonucleotides, Taq polymerase and other PCR reagents (Rechitsky et al., 1991). It was suggested that all reagents should be tested for contamination and for their ability to amplify DNA prior to their use in preconception and preimplantation diagnostic procedures, so that decontamination procedures can be applied to eliminate low level DNA contamination. As mentioned in Chapter 7, this volume, in order to minimize the chance of contamination with extraneous DNA, the establishment of a separate laboratory for preimplantation diagnosis should be considered; such a laboratory would have its own equipment and strict rules of procedure.

One of the important sources of contamination in blastomere analysis is cellular in origin. Contamination from cumulus cells, spermatozoa, polar bodies, or cell fragments might be amplified together with the blastomeres and give rise to false diagnoses. Experience has already demonstrated the difficulties of avoiding these sources of contamination: false negative diagnoses have been observed in PGD of X-linked disorders, as well as in PGD of cystic fibrosis (Soussis et al., 1991; Verlinsky et al., 1991).

Another important problem both in preconception and preimplantation genetic analysis arises with the failure of amplification, which may be as high as 5% to 15% in PCR analysis of single cells (Cui et al., 1990; Strom et al., 1991). This might be due to the actual failure of amplification of the allele present in the tube to a detectable level, or due to the failure to deposit the biopsied blastomere into the PCR reaction tube. To sort out the above failures from false negative diagnoses, internal controls have been developed based on the simultaneous amplification of two or more loci (Strom et al, 1991; Kontogianni et al., 1991). The percentage of successful amplification appears to be significantly increased with the use of nested amplification (described in Chapter 7, this volume).

A recent comprehensive analysis of possible diagnostic errors in preconception and preimplantation genetic diagnosis has been reported by Arnheim et al. (1991), based on their extensive experience in PCR analysis of single sperm. Three types of error have been considered:

1. The efficiency of the allele being amplified.
2. The probability of contamination.
3. The probability that a single cell is actually being deposited into the tube.

Authors divided the effects of these errors into three categories, reflecting varying degrees of severity. The acceptable errors were referred to as those that result in using an embryo or an oocyte that should have been used anyway, or in not using one which should have been rejected. The undesirable but tolerable errors were considered to be those that lead to not using an embryo that was rejected after being mistakenly diagnosed as affected. The most serious, unacceptable errors were the ones resulting in the transfer of an affected embryo, wrongly diagnosed as unaffected. The approximate probability of each type of error has been calculated, and this might be very useful in implementing PCR analysis in single cells for research, and possibly in PGD.

Embryo Recovery and Pregnancy Outcome Following Preconception and Preimplantation Diagnosis

PGD can be achieved either through uterine lavage after natural conception, or through IVF. The embryo obtained by uterine lavage is already at the blastocyst stage, so the only possible approach to PGD in this case may be a trophectoderm biopsy, which, as mentioned, has not yet been explored to the extent necessary for practical application. All presently available experience with PGD is based on IVF programs. These provide an appropriate framework for obtaining biopsied material from gametes and preembryos, and enough time for genetic analysis of this material so that unaffected embryos can be transferred during the initial cycle. This prompt transfer avoids freezing of the embryos, which could result in a lower implantation rate.

Unfortunately, the efficiency of IVF is not high even when micromanipulation and biopsy of gametes and preembryos, the key procedures in performing PGD, are not involved. The success rate has been reported to be as low as 15% per embryo, even in the best hands (Walters et al., 1985). Actually, the rate is much lower; for example, according to the Fifth Report of the Interim Licensing Authority for Human IVF and Embryology (1990), it ranges from 8.6% to 10% in the United Kingdom, with the differences in the percentages of the live births being related to the experience level of IVF centers involved (from 5.7% to 9.7%). Data from the American Fertility Society (1992) show a 14% delivery rate for the calendar year 1990.

In this regard, an example from the Center of Reproductive Medicine in Brussels, which is one of the most experienced centers at present, may be of particular interest (Van Steirteghem et al., 1991). The pregnancy rate per started cycle, from 1,459 oocyte retrievals in the Brussels center in 1990, was reported to be as high as 26.2% (including the pregnancies obtained after replacement of frozen, and subsequently thawed, supernumerary embryos). However, taking into consideration the well-known fact that up to one-third of fetuses are lost after implantation in any case, the authors have estimated a take-home baby rate of about 18% per cycle, one of the highest reported at the moment.

As mentioned, analysis of the factors involved in preimplantation and postimplantation fetal losses might be of great value in assessing the safety and improving the efficiency of PGD. The only data which give some guess about human embryonic loss before implantation are the early reports by Hertig and Rock. The other relevant information was reported by Gropp (1975), and Dyban and Baranov (1987) who analyzed mouse data obtained by utilizing double heterozygotes for Robertsonian translocations. Although these data do not make it possible to estimate the extent of preimplantation loss in humans, it seems possible that, as demonstrated in mice, some genetic abnormalities, such as nullisomies, haploids and some monosomies, might not be compatible with human zygote implantation. However, as the human genome seems to be activated later than the mouse genome, and since early human preimplantation development is dependent to a greater extent on the maternal gene activity than is that of the mouse, most human embryos may survive implantation and lead to positive beta human chorionic gonadotropin (-HCG) detection.

A comprehensive estimate of loss rates after implantation has been recently presented by Simpson (1991). Overall, the human loss rate after -HCG detection was evaluated to be no greater than 30%; at least half of these losses may not be recognized clinically, as they occur during the fourth gestational week, so the loss rate of only 16% could be registered about one month after menses. Analyzing the outcomes of pregnancies in about 1,000 IVF cycles, Levy et al. (1991) suggested that the group of preclinical abortions is not homogenous. About half of these pregnancies terminated 2 weeks after embryo transfer with -HCG values not higher than 21mIU/ml (chemical abortions), while the other half terminated spontaneously 4 weeks after embryo transfer (2 weeks after a missed period) with higher values of -HCG and for a longer period (called peri-implantation abortions). These preclinical abortions were suggested to be different entities, as the authors found a better prognosis for future fertility in the case of chemical (menstrual) abortions.

However, the above data on the pregnancy rate or on the take-home baby rate are based on the IVF experience, which includes mainly couples suffering from long-standing infertility, and might not be representative of the possible outcome of pregnancies following PGD. The data by Handyside et al. (1990), already mentioned, suggest that the pregnancy efficiency rate may actually be not lower, but even higher, than in IVF, as a result of the fact that most of the patients undergoing IVF for PGD do not suffer infertility and are actually much younger than IVF patients in general. Therefore, more data are needed before further considerations can be made on pregnancy outcomes in connection with PGD.

References

Arnheim N, Li H, Cui X, Navidi W (1991): Single sperm PCR analysis — implications for preimplantation genetic disease diagnosis. In Verlinsky Y, Kuliev AM (eds): "Preimplantation Genetics." New York: Plenum Press, pp. 121–130.

Bacchus C, Buselmaier W (1988): Blastomere karyotyping and transfer of chromosomally selected embryos. Hum Genet 80:333–336.

Bianchi DW, Flint AF, Pizzimenti MF, Knoll JF, Latt SA (1990): Isolation of fetal DNA from nucleated erythrocytes in maternal blood. Proc Natl Acad Sci U S A 87:3279–3283.

Bongso A, Ng SC, Lim J, Fong CY, Ratnam S (1991): Preimplantation genetics: Chromosomes of fragmented human embryos. Fertil Steril 56:66–70.

Braude P (1991): Preimplantation diagnosis of genetic disease using enzyme assays. In Verlinsky Y, Kuliev AM (eds): "Preimplantation Genetics." New York: Plenum Press, pp. 113–119.

Braude PR, Monk M, Pickering SJ, Cant A, Johnson MH (1989): Measurement of HPRT activity in the human unfertilized oocyte and pre-embryo. Prenat Diag 9:839-850.

Braude PR, Bolton VN, Moore S (1988): Human gene expression first occurs between the four- and eight- cell stages of preimplantation development. Nature 332:459–461.

Braude PR, Pelham HRB, Flalch G, Lobatto R (1979): Post transcriptional control in the early mouse embryo. Nature 282:102–105.

Coutelle C, Williams C, Handyside A, Hardy K, Winston R, Williamson R (1989): Genetic analysis of DNA from single human oocytes — a model for preimplantation diagnosis of cystic fibrosis. Br Med J 299:22–24.

Cui X, Li H, Goradia TM, Lange K, Kazazian HH, Galas DJ, Arnheim N (1990): Single sperm typing: Determination of genetic distance between the G-gamma-globin and parathyroid hormone loci. Proc Natl Acad Sci U S A 867:9389–9393.

Cui X, Li H, Goradia TM, Lange K, Kazazian HH, Galas DJ, Arnheim N (1989): Single sperm typing: Determination of genetic distance between the G-gamma globin and parathyroid hormone loci. Proc Natl Acad Sci U S A 86:9389–9393.

Dyban AP, Baranov VS (1987): "Cytogenetics of Mammalian Embryonic Development." Oxford: Oxford University Press.

Epstein CJ (1985): Mouse monosomies and trisomies as experimental systems for studying mammalian aneuploidy. Trends Genet 1:129–134.

Flach G, Johnson M, Braude P, Taylor R, Bolton V (1982): The transition from maternal to embryonic control in the 2-cell mouse embryo. EMBO J 1:681–686.

Grifo JA, Ward DC, Boyle A (1991): In situ hybridization of blastomeres from embryo biopsy. In Verlinsky Y, Kuliev AM (eds): "Preimplantation Genetics." New York: Plenum Press, pp 147–152.

Gropp A (1975): Chromosomal animal model of human disease. Fetal trisomy and development failure. In Berry L, Poswillo DE (eds): "Teratology." Berlin: Springer-Verlag, p. 17.

Handyside AH, Pattinson JK, Penketh RJA, Delhanty JDA, Winston RML, Tuddenham EDG (1989): Biopsy of human preimplantation embryos and sexing by DNA amplification. Lancet 1:347–349.

Handyside AH, Kontogiannni EH, Hardy K, Winston RML (1990): Pregnancies from biopsied human preimplantation embryos sexed by Y-specific DNA amplification. Nature 344:768–770.

Kola I, Wilton L (1991): Preimplantation embryo biopsy: Detection of trisomy in a single biopsied from a four-cell mouse embryo. Mol Reprod Develop 29:16–21.

Kontogianni EH, Hardy K, Handyside AH (1991): Coamplification of X- and Y-specific sequences for sexing preimplantation human embryos. In Verlinsky Y, Kuliev AM (eds): "Preimplantation Genetics." New York: Plenum Press pp. 139–145.

Levy T, Goldman JH, Dicker D, Ashkenazi J, Feldberg D (1991): Very early pregnancy wastage in in vitro Fertilization and embryo transfer. JIVF and Embryo Transfer. 8:250–253.

Li H, Gyllensten UB, Cui X, Saiki RK, Erlich HA, Arnheim N (1988): Amplification and analysis of DNA sequences in single human sperm and diploid cells. Nature 335:414–417.

Medical Research International, the Society for Assisted Reproductive Technology (SART) (1992): In vitro fertilization/embryo transfer in the United States: 1990 results from the IVF-ET registry. Fertil Steril 57:15–24.

Modlinsky J, McLaren A (1980): A method for visualizing the chromosomes of the second polar body of the mouse egg. J Embryol Exp Morph 60:93–97.

Monk M, Muggleton-Harris AL, Rawlings E, Whittingham DG (1988): Preimplantation diagnosis of HPRT-deficient male and carrier female mouse embryos by trophectoderm biopsy. Human Reprod 3:377–381.

Monk M, Holding C (1990): Amplification of β-haemoglobin sequence in individual human oocytes and polar bodies. Lancet 335:985.

Plachot M, Mandelbaum J, Junca AM, Grouchy J, de Salat-Baroux J, Cohen J (1989): Cytogenetic analysis and developmental capacity of normal and abnormal embryos after IVF. Human Reprod 4 (Suppl):99–103.

Plachot M, Junca AM, Mandelbaum J, Grouchy J, Salat-Baroux J, Cohen J (1987): Chromosome investigation in early life. II. Human preimplantation embryos. Hum Reprod 2:29–35.

Porter-Jordan K, Garrett CT (1990): Source of contamination in polymerase chain assay. Lancet 235:1220.

Rechitsky S, Enriquez G, Strom C (1991): DNA analysis of gametes and embryos: Analysis of delta-F508 cystic fibrosis mutation in single cells. In Verlinsky Y, Kuliev AM (eds): "Preimplantation Genetics." New York: Plenum Press, pp. 305–312.

Sermon K, Lissens W, Van Steirteghem AC, Liebaers I (1992): Enzyme expression in preimplantation embryos. Abstract of International Symposium on Preimplantation Genetics and Assisted Fertilization. Feb. 21 and 22:2. Brussels, Center for Reproductive Medicine at University of Brussels. The European Society of Human Reproduction and Embryology.

Severova EL, Dyban AP (1984): Selection of mice embryos in living condition according to sex and peculiarities of karyotype. Sov J Dev Biol Ontogenesis 15(6):585–591.

Simpson JL (1991): Assessing loss rates in the preimplantation stages of gestation. In Verlinsky Y, Kuliev AM (eds): "Preimplantation Genetics." New York: Plenum Press, pp. 175–180.

Soussis I, Jeer HS, Packham C, Margara RA, Handyside AH, Winston RML (1991): Ultrasonic and biochemical parameters of early pregnancies following transfer of biopsied human embryos for X-linked genetic disorders. 7th World Congress on In Vitro Fertilization and Assisted Procreation. Human Reprod 6(suppl 1):138.

Strom CM, Enriquez G, Rechitsky S (1991): Preimplantation genetic analysis using PCR. In Verlinsky Y, Kuliev AM (eds): "Preimplantation Genetics." New York: Plenum Press, pp. 131–138.

Strom CM, Verlinsky Y, Rechitsky S, Evsikov S, Cieslak J, Lifchez A, Valle J, Moise J, Ginsberg N, Applebaum M (1990): Preconception genetic diagnosis for cystic fibrosis by polar body removal and DNA analysis. Lancet 336:306–308.

Tesarik J, Kopecny V, Plachot M, Mandelbaum J (1988): Early morphological signs of embryonic genome expression in human preimplantation development as revealed by quantitative electron microscopy. Dev Biol 128:15–20

Van Steirteghem A, Liu J, Van den Abbeel E, Liebaers I, Devroey P (1991): In Verlinsky Y, Kuliev AM (eds): "Preimplantation Genetics." New York: Plenum Press, pp. 155–164.

Verlinsky Y, Pergament E, Binor Z, Rawlins R (1987): Genetic analysis of human embryos prior to implantation: Future applications of in-vitro fertilization in treatment and prevention of human genetic diseases. In Ferchlinger W and Kemeter P (eds): "Future Aspects in Human In-Vitro Fertilization." Berlin: Springer-Verlag, pp. 262–266.

Verlinsky Y, Rechitsky S, Cieslak J, Evsikov S, Lifchez A, Valle J, Ginsberg N, White M, Strom C (1991): Reliability of preconception and preimplantation genetic diagnosis. Proceedings of the 8th International Congress of Human Genetics.Am J Hum Genet (suppl)49,4:22.

Walters DE, Edwards RG, Meistrich ML (1985): A statistical evaluation of implantation after replacing one or more human embryos. J Reprod Fertil 74:557–563.

CHAPTER 10

Ethical Issues

Anver M. Kuliev

Considerations on ethical issues are evolving along with the evolution of technology for the control of genetic diseases, and have now become one of the key subjects in discussing the acceptability of preconception and preimplantation diagnosis of genetic disorders. Ethical and legal issues will determine to a considerable extent whether these new approaches will be promoted as an integral part of preventive genetics services, or will be waived on ethical grounds (The Ethics Committee of The American Fertility Society, 1990; Kuliev and Modell, 1991). Preimplantation genetic diagnosis (PGD) could be regarded as an ethically acceptable procedure in the context of the general objective of genetics services, which, according to WHO, is to help genetically disadvantaged people to live and reproduce as normally and as responsibly as possible (WHO, 1985). As PGD is heavily based on IVF it is relevant to mention that IVF is considered to be ethically acceptable in many countries (Walters, 1987; Milunsky, 1991). However, many ethical and legal issues are still very complicated and are confronted differently, even in various states in one country (Robertson, 1991). Nevertheless, having analyzed existing differences in current legal restrictions in this field in the United States, Robertson et al. (1991) came to the conclusion that selection of preembryos on genetic grounds is ethically acceptable, since the goal of avoiding the birth of offspring with severe genetic handicaps is a constitutional right of procreative liberty.

Because PGD is currently at the very early experimental stage, its future will depend to a great extent upon the legalization of human embryo research in general. A recent review of the ethics of human embryo research has shown that there is no national or international consensus on research into the beginning of human life (Cohen and Hotz, 1991). Comprehensive legislation to regulate emerging reproductive technology and human embryo research has been enacted in some European countries. In the United Kingdom, the "Human Fertilization and Embryology Bill" forbids embryo research except with approval of the government, and allows authorized research on human embryos during the first 14 days of development (McLaren, 1990). In Spain, the law forbids the fertilization of human oocytes for any purposes other than human procreation, but research on "preembryos" up to the 14th day of development is permitted under the supervision of national health and scientific authorities (Peinado and Russell, 1990). As in the application of other health technologies, further development and improvement of PGD will depend on the opportunity to carry out human embryonic research.

Current research in PGD has already approached the clinical trial stage, and it seems clear that separate consent forms should be developed with research protocols to be approved by institutional ethics committees. Moreover, as PGD diagnosis at the present stage could be considered as only presumptive, it would be necessary to have confirmatory CVS or amniocentesis. Clearly the future of PGD would, first of all, depend on the safety of the methods involved and the accuracy of the genetic analysis. Some of the longstanding ethical problems would probably be solved by preimplantation diagnosis; for instance, the abortion issue would be avoided as a result of this new approach. Other ethical questions could become a serious obstacle, particularly those relating to antiscience movements apprehensive about new technologies related to fetal research. These considerations are relevant to the subject of PGD, as well as to any other new method, as we proceed with further development of the appropriate technology for controlling genetic disability.

References

Cohen J, Hotz RL (1991): Human embryo research: Ethics and recent progress. Curr Opin Obstet Gynecol 3:678–684.

Kuliev AM, Modell B (1991): Ethical issues in the control of genetic diseases. In Verlinsky Y, Kuliev AM (eds): "Preimplantation Genetics." New York: Plenum Press, pp. 233–244.

McLaren A (1990): Research on the human conceptus and its regulation in Britain today. J Royal Soc Med 344:768–770.

Milunsky A (1991): Ethical and selected medical aspects of preimplantation genetic diagnosis. In Verlinsky Y, Kuliev AM (eds): "Preimplantation Genetics." New York: Plenum Press, pp. 245–252.

Peinado JA, Russell SE (1990): The Spanish care governing assisted reproduction techniques: A summary. Hum Reprod 5:634–636.

Robertson J (1991): Legal and ethical issues in preimplantation genetic diagnosis. In Verlinsky Y, Kuliev AM (eds): "Preimplantation Genetics." New York: Plenum Press, pp. 253–269.

The Ethics Committee of the American Fertility Society: Ethics and the new reproductive technologies (1990): Fertil Steril 53(Suppl 2):5–15.

Walters L (1987): Ethics and new reproductive technologies: An international review of committee statements. Hastings Center Report 17:3–22.

WHO (1985): Community approaches to the control of hereditary diseases. Report of a WHO Advisory Group. Unpublished WHO document. HDP/WG/85.10. (Can be obtained free of charge from Hereditary Diseases Progeamme, WHO, Geneva, Switzerland).

CHAPTER 11

Conclusion

Yury Verlinsky and Anver M. Kuliev

Although introduction of a first trimester prenatal diagnosis by CVS has considerably improved the possibility for prevention of genetic diseases, it requires a selective abortion in case of an affected fetus. Preimplantation genetic diagnosis (PGD) has been initiated to provide the option of avoiding the birth of an affected child without the need for abortion as an obligatory component in the control program. This book has described these important developments with the emphasis on addressing existing problems to be solved before PGD can be practically applied.

At present two approaches for PGD have been realized: (1) polar body removal (PBR) for preconception genetic diagnosis and (2) blastomere biopsy for preembryo diagnosis of genetic disease. Both of these approaches become possible due to the progress in micromanipulation and biopsy, and in genetic analysis of single cells by PCR. The use of both of these approaches has already demonstrated the feasibility of preconception and preimplantation diagnosis of genetic disorders, but has also raised important problems to be studied in the future.

One such problem is the possibility of DNA contamination and allele-specific PCR failure in analyzing the DNA of a single cell, which can lead to diagnostic errors and can require specially designed research. The other challenge is enzyme analysis in preembryos, which is not reliable at the moment. An even greater challenge is PGD of chromosomal disorders, as cytogenetic analysis is needed not only for couples at high risk for chromosomal abnormalities, but also to exclude possible cytogenetic disturbances either in couples who have been referred in order to avoid genetic disorders or even in IVF patients. Because of the high frequency of chromosomal abnormalities in early pregnancy, the introduction of preimplantation cytogenetic analysis could considerably improve the current limited embryo recovery and pregnancy outcome that follow preconception and preimplantation diagnosis, as well as those in the general IVF programs.

Although, in the future, the indications for PGD might be, in principle, the same as those for prenatal diagnosis (with the above mentioned exceptions), at present they should obviously be limited to couples at high risk for having a child with genetic disorders, who cannot accept prenatal diagnosis followed by elective abortion as an option. Ethical considerations are of great importance as they provide impetus for the PGD that may contribute considerably to finding more ethically acceptable approaches for the prevention of genetic disorders and to obviating the need for selective abortion in preventive services.

INDEX